# Air Fryer Oven C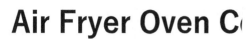

*Quick and Effortless Recipes for Health and Delicious Air Fryer*
*Homemade Meal*

## Sarah Miller

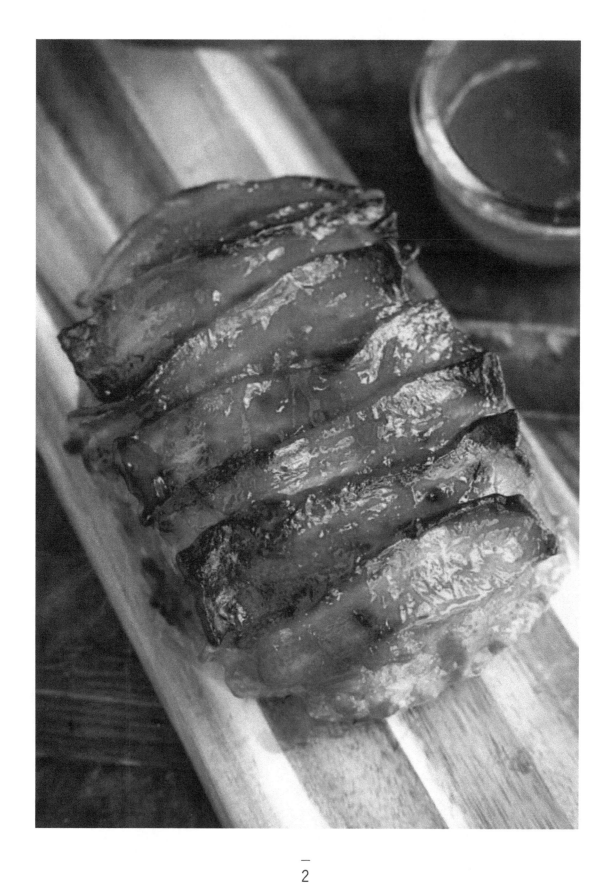

# Table of contents

*Introduction* ........................................................................................7
Chapter 1.          *Air Fryer Oven Tips & Tricks and Its Function Keys* ................9
Chapter 2.          *Recipes*.........................................................................12
SIMPLE SIRLOIN ROAST ........................................................12
HERBED CHUCK ROAST ........................................................14
SEASONED BEEF TOP ROAST.................................................15
SIMPLE BEEF TENDERLOIN .....................................................17
STRIP STEAK.......................................................................18
BACON-WRAPPED FILET MIGNON.............................................20
BEEF JERKY .......................................................................21
MEATBALLS .......................................................................24
BEEF BURGERS ...................................................................26
BEEF CASSEROLE .................................................................29
GARLICKY PORK TENDERLOIN ...............................................30
GLAZED PORK TENDERLOIN ...................................................32
BUTTERED PORK LOIN..........................................................33
SPICY PORK SHOULDER.........................................................35
BBQ PORK RIBS .................................................................37
CHEESEBURGER EGG ROLLS ....................................................39
AIR FRIED GRILLED STEAK .....................................................41
JUICY CHEESEBURGERS .........................................................42
BEEF BRISKET RECIPE FROM TEXAS ..........................................44
COPYCAT TACO BELL CRUNCH WRAPS .....................................46
STEAK AND MUSHROOM GRAVY .............................................48
CHIMICHURRI SKIRT STEAK....................................................50
COUNTRY FRIED STEAK.........................................................53
CREAMY BURGER & POTATO BAKE..........................................55
BEEFY 'N CHEESY SPANISH RICE CASSEROLE ...............................57
WARMING WINTER BEEF WITH CELERY ....................................59
BEEF & VEGGIE SPRING ROLLS................................................61
CHARRED ONIONS AND STEAK CUBE BBQ .................................63
BEEF STROGANOFF ..............................................................65
CHEESY GROUND BEEF AND MAC TACO CASSEROLE ....................66
HAM AND CHEESE ROLLUPS ...................................................69
PORK TAQUITOS .................................................................71
JUICY PORK RIBS OLE ...........................................................73
PORK TENDERS WITH BELL PEPPERS.........................................74
CAJUN BACON PORK LOIN FILLET ............................................76
SCOTCH EGGS.....................................................................78
ASIAN PORK CHOPS .............................................................80
BBQ RIBLETS .....................................................................81
BACON-WRAPPED STUFFED PORK CHOPS...................................83
PANKO-BREADED PORK CHOPS................................................85
CAJUN PORK STEAKS.............................................................87
PORCHETTA-STYLE PORK CHOPS .............................................88
DRY RUB BABY BACK RIBS .....................................................90
PORK MILANESE ..................................................................91

ROASTED PORK TENDERLOIN .................................................................... 94

JUICY PORK CHOPS .............................................................................. 96

CRISPY MEATBALLS ............................................................................. 98

FLAVOURFUL STEAK ............................................................................. 100

LEMON GARLIC LAMB CHOPS ................................................................. 102

HONEY MUSTARD PORK TENDERLOIN ......................................................... 104

EASY ROSEMARY LAMB CHOPS ............................................................... 106

JUICY STEAK BITES ............................................................................ 107

GREEK LAMB CHOPS ........................................................................... 109

EASY BEEF ROAST ............................................................................. 111

HERB BUTTER RIB-EYE STEAK ................................................................ 113

BBQ PORK CHOPS ............................................................................. 115

SIMPLE BEEF PATTIES ........................................................................ 117

MARINATED PORK CHOPS ..................................................................... 118

PORK SATAY .................................................................................... 120

PORK BURGERS WITH RED CABBAGE SALAD ............................................... 122

CRISPY MUSTARD PORK TENDERLOIN ....................................................... 124

ESPRESSO-GRILLED PORK TENDERLOIN ..................................................... 126

PORK AND POTATOES ......................................................................... 128

LIGHT HERBED MEATBALLS ................................................................... 131

BROWN RICE AND BEEF-STUFFED BELL PEPPERS ......................................... 133

BEEF AND BROCCOLI .......................................................................... 136

BEEF AND FRUIT STIR-FRY ................................................................... 138

BEEF RISOTTO .................................................................................. 140

# Introduction

This Air fryer Oven Cookbook contains easy, delicious, and healthy recipes that can be prepared within few minutes. It is highly recommended for people with busy schedules and also for those on the Weight Watchers Program.

Even if you have never tried the Air Fryer Oven before, it promises you one thing, after having this cookbook, you will be kicking yourself for having not discovered this sooner.

It will inspire you to clean up your kitchen from all the useless appliances that clutter your countertop and start putting the Air Fryer Oven to good use. The air fryer oven will give you lots of joy, time, and, most importantly, tasty dishes. Feel free to adjust and alter these recipes, or simply use them as a springboard of inspiration for your own creations!

The Air Fryer Oven is definitely a change in lifestyle that will make things much easier for you and your family. You'll discover increased energy, decreased hunger, a boosted metabolism, and of course, a LOT of free time! You will know that it is not just a simple kitchen appliance. Still, it's truly a kitchen-miracle that will bring relief and satisfaction with its user-friendly functions, time plus energy-effective heating method, and multiple cooking options. This cookbook will share as many different recipes to provide an extensive guideline to all the frequent oven users. With the latest air fryer oven functions, you can air fry, dehydrate, broil, toast, roast, and bake all kinds of the dishes. Please give it a full read and find out tons of new ways to add more colors and flavors to your dinner table using the Air fryer Oven.

**Why Use an Air Fryer Oven?**

First and foremost, the air fryer oven became popular for its numerous health benefits. The convenience and ease of using an air fryer oven give an effortless choice for people that wants a healthy and delicious meal in a matter of time. For those who are hesitant on the air fryer oven potential and favor the conventional cooking way, perhaps the following benefits are enough to assure them to make the switch to efficient cooking:

- Great for cooking solidified foods without oil and extraordinary or pre-heating foods.

- Because of littler bins, the food cooked speedier when contrasted with ovens, and no pre-heating is fundamental.

- The kind of food is brilliant because the heat gives a pleasantly fresh and does not burn.

- Perfect for two individuals or littler segments. There's such a significant number of greater models out there to cook bigger parts for multiple individuals. The potential outcomes are inestimable.

- It's a healthier method of cooking fried or crispy foods. In general, you can utilize substantially less oil to accomplish crunchy and crispy finished foods.

- There's tidy little up and less splattering of oil while cooking. Everything gets contained pleasantly inside the air fryer while cooking.

- Food cooks fresh due to the littler cooking zone, and the heating component is nearer to the food.

- There's no need to warm up your home in summer when you're longing for something warm, roasted, or pan-fried.

**Cleaning and Maintenance**

Remember to clean your air fryer oven and accessories according to the instructions and safety precautions after each cooking adventure. Like every appliance, maintenance is needed to get what you would like in the device. Any tool employed for preparing food must be stored spotlessly clean. Don't let dirt develop and clean the environment fryer frequently, so you get great results when you make use of the air fryer oven. You have to make sure you remember it, "keep clean and maintain it" for best results efficiently because taken care of the appliance will always last longer. We provide you with some cleaning tips; however, it is not difficult. The outdoors and inside parts could be cleaned relatively easily and ought to be done frequently. Within the situation from the heating coil, get it done a couple of occasions annually only.

With so many recipes and a comprehensive guideline about the air fryer oven, you will know how to put to its best use and enjoy a range of flavorsome crispy meals in no time. This ten in one multipurpose kitchen miracle has brought much-wanted peace and comfort to the homemakers' lives who can now cook a healthy and delicious meal for their family in no time. This cookbook's different segment provides a step-by-step direction to cook various meals ranging from breakfast, poultry, meat, vegetables, snacks, and much more. Get this latest hit Air Fryer Oven Cookbook and bring convenience to your kitchen floor now. If you had an air fryer oven and you don't know what to cook in it, now you do – with all the recipes at its best!

What are you still waiting for? Start cooking in your air fryer oven and enjoy all the foods you thought were not healthy!

# Chapter 1. **Air Fryer Oven Tips & Tricks and Its Function Keys**

Air fryer Ovens are designed to be super easy to use. Here's a little tip to get you started:

## Choosing A Recipe

Choose a recipe that you can cook in your air fryer. Remember that most foods you cook in your microwave or oven, or on the stovetop, can be prepared in the air fryer – except for those recipes with a lot of fat or liquids. You can use my air fryer cookbook to help you find suitable recipes.

## Preparing the Air Fryer

Read through the recipe to the end, so you know what accessories you need for cooking. Some recipes call for using the basket, rack, or rotisserie that comes with the air fryer. Other recipes use cake or muffin pans that you can insert into the air fryer. Just be sure these pans fit into the fryer and are safe to use.

## Preparing the Ingredients

Gather the ingredients for the recipe and prep them according to the instructions. When prepped, put the ingredients into the air fryer or in the basket, rack, or pans within the air fryer. Use parchment baking paper or a light mist of oil spray to prevent food from sticking.

Never crowd food in the air fryer or over-fill. Food that is crowded in the air fryer won't cook evenly and can be raw and under-cooked. If you're preparing for a crowd, you may have to cook more than one batch.

## Setting the Temperature and Time

Check the recipe for the correct temperature and time setting. You can set manually; you can use the digital setting for the temperature and time needed for the recipe. Most air fryers also have preset functions that make it easy to set according to each recipe.

## Check Food During Cooking

Many air fryer oven recipes require you to check the food while cooking so that it cooks evenly and doesn't over-cook. You will need to shake, flip, or toss the food to distribute it. Or for some recipes, you'll need to turn the food about halfway through when cooking so that it cooks and crisps all the way thoroughly.

## Cleaning the Air Fryer

Once the food is cooked, remove and unplug the air fryer. Let it cool completely before cleaning. Follow the directions that come with the air fryer oven for proper cleaning. Never scrub or use abrasive cleaners when cleaning the fryer or the fryer accessories.

## Using the Basket or Rack

Some air fryers use a round basket where foods are cooked, while other models will have layered racks that fit into a square cooking space, much like a small oven. Most of the recipes given in this cookbook can be used for both baskets and racks.

## Keep an Eye on Timing

You'll find that air fryers cook at different temperatures depending on what model you have. It is why it's essential to check on foods during the cooking process, so you don't over or undercook them. If you've cut back on quantities in some of the recipes, be sure to cut the cooking time down accordingly. Remember, hints are just recommendations to guide you as you use your air fryer.

## Using Oil Sprays

Most of the recipes use an oil spray. But if you desire, you can use any brand you want. Or make your own by merely putting olive oil into a small spray bottle. Use a small amount of oil and spray over the basket and trays to prevent food from sticking. Some of the recipes require you to spray the food with oil directly.

## Function Keys

The following are the functions keys of an Air Fryer Oven:

## Play/Pause Button

This Play/Pause button allows you to pause during the middle of the cooking so you can shake the air fryer basket or flip the food to ensure it cooks evenly.

## -/+ Button /Minus or Plus Button

This button is used to change the time or temperature.

## Keep Warm

This function keeps your food warm for 30 minutes.

## Food Presets

This button gives you the ability to cook food without second-guessing. The time and temperature are already set, so new users find this setting useful.

## Roast or Broil

You can roast or broil with this setting. When using a conventional oven, you need to brown the meat before roasting. You can skip this step when cooking with an air fryer.

## Dehydrate

This setting cooks and dries food at a low temperature for a few hours. With this option, you can create your beef jerky or dried fruit.

# Chapter 2.   **Recipes**

## Simple Sirloin Roast

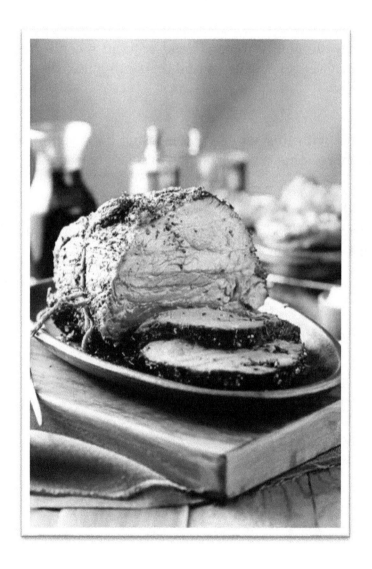

Preparation time: 15 minutes

Cooking time: 50 minutes

Servings: 8

**Ingredients:**

Sirloin roast – 2½ lb.

Salt and ground black pepper

**Directions:**

Rub the roast with salt and black pepper generously. Insert the rotisserie rod through the roast, one on each side of the rod.

Select "Roast" at 350 °F. Set the time for 50 minutes and press "Start."

When it's done, press the red lever to release the rod.

Place the roast onto a platter for about 10 minutes before slicing. Cut the sirloin roast into desired-sized slices and serve.

**Nutrition:**

Calories 258

Carbs 0g

Fat 11.8g

Protein 37.9g

# Herbed Chuck Roast

Preparation time: 15 minutes

Cooking time: 45 minutes

Servings: 5

**Ingredients:**

2 lbs. Beef chuck roast

1 tbsp Olive oil

1 tsp Dried rosemary, crushed

1 tsp dried thyme, crushed

Salt, as required

**Directions:**

In a bowl, add the oil, herbs, and salt and mix well. Coat the beef roast with herb mixture generously. Arrange the beef roast onto the greased cooking tray.

Select "Air Fry" to 360 °F. Set the time for 45 minutes and press "Start."

Remove and place the roast onto a cutting board.

With a piece of foil, cover the beef roast for about 20 minutes before slicing. With a sharp knife, cut the beef roast into desired-sized slices and serve.

**Nutrition:**

Calories 32

Carbs 0.3g

Fat 14.2g

Protein 55.1g

# Seasoned Beef Top Roast

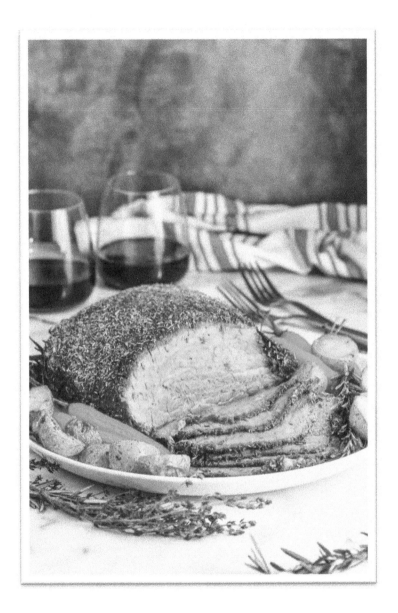

Preparation time: 15 minutes

Cooking time: 45 minutes

Servings: 5

**Ingredients:**

3 lb. Beef top roast

1 tbsp Olive oil

2 tbsp Montreal steak seasoning

**Directions:**

Coat the roast with oil and then rub with the seasoning generously. With kitchen twines, tie the roast to keep it compact. Arrange the roast onto the cooking tray.

Select "Air Fry" over 360 F. Set the time for 45 minutes

Remove and place the roast onto a platter for about 10 minutes before slicing. Slice into desired-sized slices and serve.

**Nutrition:**

Calories 269

Carbs 0g

Fat 9.9g

Protein 41.3g

# Simple Beef Tenderloin

Preparation time: 15 minutes

Cooking time: 40 minutes

Servings: 4

**Ingredients:**

1 (3-lb.) Beef tenderloin, trimmed

2 tbsps. Olive oil

Salt and ground black pepper

**Directions:**

Rub tenderloin with oil and then season with salt and black pepper evenly. Arrange the tenderloin onto the greased cooking tray.

Select "Bake" and then adjust the temperature to 400 °F. Set the time for 40 minutes and press "Start."

Remove, then place the tenderloin onto a cutting board. With a piece of foil, cover the tenderloin for about 10 minutes before slicing. With a sharp knife, cut the tenderloin into desired-sized slices and serve.

**Nutrition:**

Calories 380

Carbs 0g

Fat 19.1g

Protein 49.2g

# Strip Steak

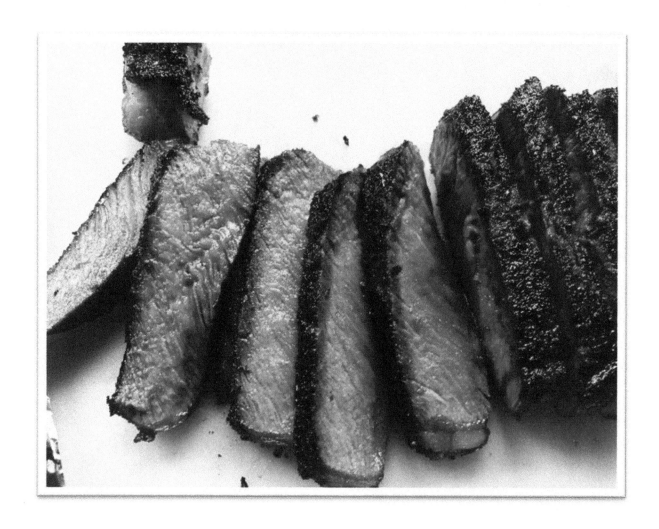

Preparation time: 15 minutes

Cooking time: 8 minutes

Servings: 2

**Ingredients:**

9½-oz. New York strip steak

Salt and ground black pepper

1 tsp Olive oil

**Directions:**

Coat the steak with oil and then sprinkle with salt and black pepper evenly. Arrange the steak onto the greased cooking tray.

Arrange the pan in the bottom of the air fryer oven, then select "Air Fry" to 400 °F.

Set the time for 8 minutes and press "Start."

Remove, then place the steak onto a platter for about 10 minutes. Cut the steak into desired-sized slices and serve immediately.

**Nutrition:**

Calories 344

Carbs 0g

Fat 22.5g

Protein 36g

# Bacon-Wrapped Filet Mignon

Preparation time: 15 minutes

Cooking time: 15 minutes

Servings: 2

**Ingredients:**

2 Bacon slices

2 Filet mignons

Salt and ground black pepper

Olive oil cooking spray

**Directions:**

Wrap 1 bacon slice around each filet mignon and secure with toothpicks. Season the fillets with the salt and black pepper lightly.

Arrange the filet mignon onto a rack and spray with cooking spray.

Select "Air Fry" to 375 °F. Set the time for 15 minutes and press "Start."

When it shows "Turn Food," turn the filets. Remove, then serve hot.

**Nutrition:**

Calories 360

Carbs 0.4g

Fat 19.6g

Protein 42.6g

# Beef Jerky

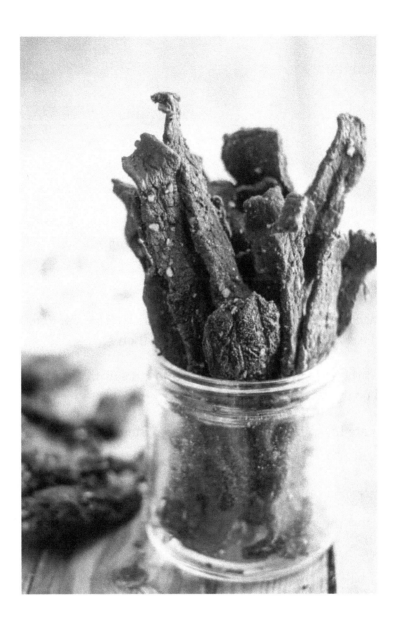

Preparation time: 15 minutes

Cooking time: 3 hours

Servings: 4

**Ingredients:**

1½ lbs. Beef round, trimmed

½ cup Worcestershire sauce

½ cup Low-sodium soy sauce

2 tsp Honey

1 tsp Liquid smoke

2 tsp Onion powder

½ tsp Red pepper flakes, crushed

Ground black pepper

**Directions:**

In a zip-top bag, place the beef and freeze for 1-2 hours to firm up. Place the beef meat onto a cutting board and cut against the grain into 1/8-¼-inch strips.

In a large bowl, add the remaining ingredients and mix until thoroughly combined. Add the steak slices and coat with the mixture generously.

Refrigerate to marinate for about 4-6 hours. Remove the beef slices from the bowl and with paper towels; pat dries them.

Divide the steak strips onto the cooking trays and arrange them in an even layer.

Select "Dehydrate" and then adjust the temperature to 160 °F. Set the time for 3 hours and press "Start."

Once it shows "Add Food," insert 1 tray in the top position and another in the center position.

After 1½ hours, switch the position of cooking trays. Remove the trays, then serve.

**Nutrition:**

Calories 372

Carbs 12g

Fat 10.7g

Protein 53.8g

# Meatballs

Preparation time: 15 minutes

Cooking time: 30 minutes

Servings: 8

**Ingredients:**

For Meatballs:

2 lb. Lean ground beef

2/3 cup Quick-cooking oats

½ cup Ritz crackers, crushed

1 can Evaporate milk

2 large eggs, beaten lightly

1 tsp Honey

1 tbsp Dried onion, minced

1 tsp Garlic powder

1 tsp ground cumin

Salt and ground black pepper

For Sauce:

1/3 cup Orange marmalade

1/3 cup Honey

1/3 cup Brown sugar

2 tbsp Cornstarch

2 tbsp Soy sauce

1-2 tbsp Hot sauce

1 tbsp Worcestershire sauce

**Directions:**

For meatballs: Add all the meatball ingredients into a bowl and mix until thoroughly combined. Make 1½-inch balls from the mixture.

Arrange half of the meatballs onto the greased cooking tray in a single layer.

Select "Air Fry" to 380 °F. Set the time for 15 minutes and press "Start."

When it shows "Turn Food," turn the meatballs. Remove, then repeat the process with the remaining meatballs.

Meanwhile, for the sauce: In a small pan, add all ingredients over medium heat and cook until thickened, stirring continuously. Serve the meatballs with the topping of sauce.

**Nutrition:**

Calories 411

Carbs 38.8g

Fat 11.1g

Protein 38.9g

# Beef Burgers

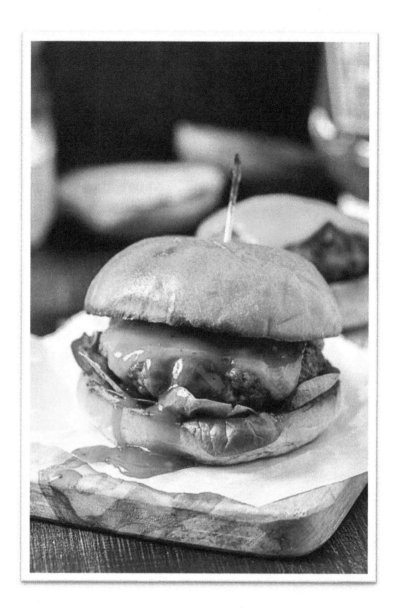

Preparation time: 15 minutes

Cooking time: 18 minutes

Servings: 4

**Ingredients:**

For Burgers:

1 lb. Ground beef

½ cup Panko breadcrumbs

¼ cup Onion, chopped finely

3 tbsps. Dijon mustard

3 tsp Low-sodium soy sauce

2 tsp fresh rosemary, minced

Salt, as required

For Topping:

2 tbsp Dijon mustard

1 tbsp Brown sugar

1 tsp Soy sauce

4 Gruyere cheese slices

**Directions:**

Add all the burger ingredients into a bowl and mix until thoroughly combined. Make 4 equal-sized patties from the mixture. Arrange the patties onto the greased cooking tray.

Select "Air Fry" to 370 °F.

Set the time for 15 minutes and press "Start." When it shows "Add Food," insert the cooking rack in the center position. When it shows "Turn Food," turn the burgers.

Meanwhile, mix the mustard, brown sugar, and soy sauce in a small bowl to make the sauce. When done, remove and coat the burgers with the sauce.

Top each burger with 1 cheese slice. Return the tray and select "Broil." Set the time for 3 minutes and press "Start." Remove, and serve hot.

**Nutrition:**

Calories 402

Carbs 6.3g

Fat 18g

Protein 44.4g

# Beef Casserole

Preparation time: 15 minutes

Cooking time: 25 minutes

Servings: 6

**Ingredients:**

2 lbs. Ground beef

2 tbsp taco seasoning

1 cup Cheddar cheese, shredded

1 cup Cottage cheese

1 cup of salsa

**Directions:**

In a bowl, add the beef and taco seasoning and mix well. Add the cheeses and salsa and stir to combine. Place the mixture into a baking dish that will fit in the Air Fryer Oven.

Choose "Air Fry" to 370 °F.

Set the time for 25 minutes and press "Start." After that, serve warm.

**Nutrition:**

Calories 412

Carbs 6.3g

Fat 16.5g

Protein 56.4g

# Garlicky Pork Tenderloin

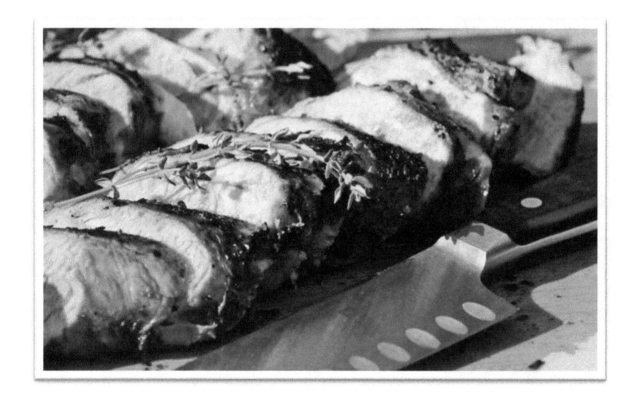

Preparation time: 15 minutes

Cooking time: 20 minutes

Servings: 5

**Ingredients:**

½ lb. Pork tenderloin

Nonstick cooking spray

2 Small heads of roasted garlic

Salt and ground black pepper

**Directions:**

Lightly spray all the sides of pork with cooking spray and then season with salt and black pepper. Now, rub the pork with roasted garlic.

Arrange the roast onto the lightly greased cooking tray.

Select "Air Fry" and the temperature to 400 °F. Set the time for 20 minutes and press "Start." When it shows "Turn Food," turn the pork.

Remove, then put the roast onto a platter for about 10 minutes before slicing. Slice and serve.

**Nutrition:**

Calories 238

Carbs 1.7g

Fat 1g

Protein 35.9g

# Glazed Pork Tenderloin

Preparation time: 15 minutes

Cooking time: 20 minutes

Servings: 3

**Ingredients:**

1 lb. Pork tenderloin

2 tbsp Sriracha

2 tbsps. Honey

Salt, as required

**Directions:**

Insert the rotisserie rod through the pork tenderloin. Put the rotisserie forks, one on each side of the rod to secure the pork tenderloin.

In a small bowl, add the Sriracha, honey, and salt and mix well. Brush the pork tenderloin with the honey mixture evenly.

Select "Air Fry" to 350 °F.

Set the timer within 20 minutes and press "Start."

When done, press the red lever to release the rod. Remove the pork and place it onto a platter for about 10 minutes before slicing. Cut the roast into desired-sized slices and serve.

**Nutrition:**

Calories 269

Carbs 13.5g

Fat 5.3g

Protein 39.7g

# Buttered Pork Loin

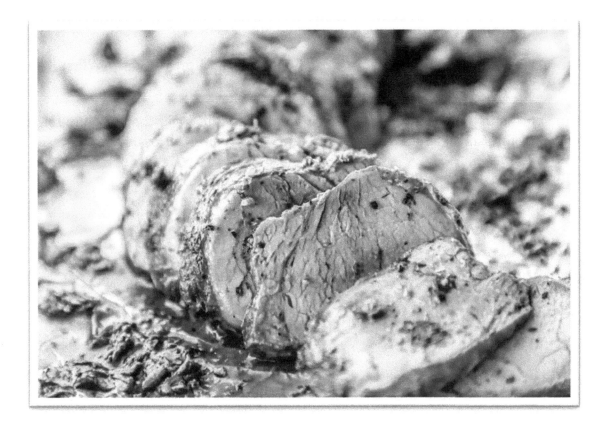

Preparation time: 15 minutes

Cooking time: 30 minutes

Servings: 6

**Ingredients:**

2 lb. Pork loin

3 tbsp butter, melted and divided

Salt and ground black pepper

**Directions:**

Arrange a wire rack in a baking dish that will fit in the Air Fryer Oven. Coat the pork loin with melted butter evenly and then rub with salt and black pepper generously.

Arrange the pork loin into the prepared baking dish.

Choose "Air Fry" to 350 °F. Set the time for 30 minutes and press "Start." When it shows "Turn Food," do not turn the food.

Place the pork loin onto a cutting board. With a piece of foil, cover the pork loin for about 10 minutes before slicing. Slice the pork loin into desired-sized slices and serve.

**Nutrition:**

Calories 417

Carbs 0g

Fat 26.8g

Protein 41.4g

# Spicy Pork Shoulder

Preparation time: 15 minutes

Cooking time: 55 minutes

Servings: 6

**Ingredients:**

1 tsp. ground cumin

1 tsp. Cayenne pepper

1 tsp. Garlic powder

Salt and ground black pepper

2 lbs. Skin-on pork shoulder

**Directions:**

In a small bowl, place spices, salt, and black pepper and mix well. Arrange the pork shoulder onto a cutting board, skin-side down.

Season the inner side of the pork shoulder with salt and black pepper. With kitchen twines, tie the pork shoulder into a long round cylinder shape.

Season the outer side of the pork shoulder with the spice mixture. Insert the rotisserie rod through the pork shoulder. Insert the rotisserie forks, one on each side of the rod to secure the pork shoulder.

Select "Roast" and then adjust the temperature to 350 °F.

Set the time for 55 minutes and press "Start." When it shows "Add Food," press the red lever down and load the rod's left side into the air fryer oven.

Now, slide the rod's left side into the groove along the metal bar, so it doesn't move. Then, close the door and touch "Rotate."

Remove the pork from the air fryer oven and place onto a platter for about 10 minutes before slicing. With a sharp knife, cut the pork shoulder into desired-sized slices and serve.

**Nutrition:**

Calories 445

Carbs 0.7g

Fat 32.5g

Protein 35.4g

# BBQ Pork Ribs

Preparation time: 15 minutes

Cooking time: 26 minutes

Servings: 4

**Ingredients:**

¼ cup Honey divided

¾ cup BBQ sauce

2 tbsps. Tomato ketchup

1 tbsp. Worcestershire sauce

1 tbsp. Soy sauce

½ tsp. Garlic powder

Ground white pepper

1¾ lbs. Pork ribs

**Directions:**

In a bowl, mix 3 tbsp of honey and the remaining ingredients except for the pork ribs. Add the pork ribs and coat with the mixture generously.

Refrigerate to marinate for about 20 minutes. Arrange the ribs onto the greased cooking tray.

Select "Air Fry" to 355 °F. Set the time for 26 minutes and press "Start."

When the display shows "Turn Food," turn the ribs. Transfer the ribs onto serving plates. Put the remaining honey and serve immediately.

**Nutrition:**

Calories 691

Carbs 37g

Fat 35.3g

Protein 53.1g

# Cheeseburger Egg Rolls

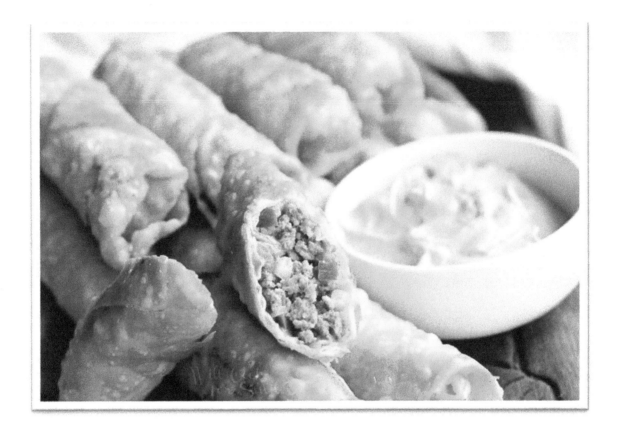

Preparation time: 10 minutes

Cooking time: 7 minutes

Servings: 6

**Ingredients:**

6 egg roll wrappers

6 chopped dill pickle chips

1 tbsp. yellow mustard

3 tbsp. cream cheese

3 tbsp. shredded cheddar cheese

½ C. chopped onion

½ C. chopped bell pepper

¼ tsp onion powder

¼ tsp. garlic powder

8 ounces of raw lean ground beef

**Directions:**

Put the seasonings, beef, onion, and bell pepper in a skillet. Mix and crumble the beef until fully cooked.

Remove, then put the cream cheese, mustard, and cheddar cheese, mixing until melted.

Put the beef mixture into a large bowl and put the pickles.

Arrange the egg wrappers, then place 1/6th of beef batter into each one. Wet the egg roll wrapper edges slightly using water. Tuck sides to the middle and seals it with water.

Repeat the process with all the remaining egg rolls.

Place rolls into the air fryer, one batch at a time.

Set temperature to 392°F, and set time to 7 minutes.  Serve.

**Nutrition:**

Calories: 148

Carbs: 0g

Fat: 0g

Protein: 0g

# Air Fried Grilled Steak

Preparation time: 5 minutes

Cooking time: 45 minutes

Servings: 2

**Ingredients:**

2 top sirloin steaks

3 tablespoons butter, melted

3 tablespoons olive oil

Salt and pepper to taste

**Directions:**

Preheat the air fryer oven for 5 minutes. Season the sirloin steaks with olive oil, salt, and pepper.

Put the beef in the air fryer basket—Cook for 45 minutes at 350°F.

Once cooked, serve with butter.

**Nutrition:**

Calories: 302

Carbs: 16g

Fat: 15g

Protein: 26g

# Juicy Cheeseburgers

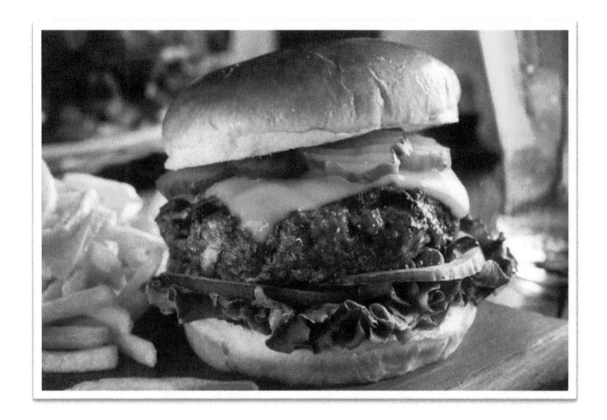

Preparation time: 5 minutes

Cooking time: 15 minutes

Servings: 4

**Ingredients:**

1 pound 93% lean ground beef

1 teaspoon Worcestershire sauce

1 tablespoon burger seasoning

Salt

Pepper

Cooking oil

4 slices cheese

buns

**Directions:**

Mix the ground beef, Worcestershire, burger seasoning, salt, and pepper to taste until well blended in a large bowl.

Grease the air fryer basket using cooking oil. You will need only a quick spritz. The burgers will produce oil as they cook. Shape the mixture into 4 patties.

Place the burgers in the air fryer. Set temperature to 375°F, and set time to 8 minutes.

Cook for 8 minutes. Flip the burgers. Cook again within 3 to 4 minutes.

Put a slice of cheese in each burger. Cook again in a minute, or until the cheese has melted. Serve on buns with any additional toppings of your choice.

**Nutrition:**

Calories: 249

Carbs: 24g

Fat: 11g

Protein: 12g

# Beef Brisket Recipe from Texas

Preparation time: 15 minutes

Cooking time: 1 hour & 30 minutes

Servings: 8

**Ingredients:**

1 ½ cup beef stock

1 bay leaf

1 tablespoon garlic powder

1 tablespoon onion powder

2 pounds beef brisket, trimmed

2 tablespoons chili powder

2 teaspoons dry mustard

4 tablespoons olive oil

Salt and pepper to taste

**Directions:**

Preheat the air fryer oven for 5 minutes. Put all the fixings in a deep baking dish that will fit in the air fryer.

Bake for 1 hour and 30 minutes at 400°F. Stir the beef every after 30 minutes to soak in the sauce.

**Nutrition:**

Calories: 170

Carbs: 0g

Fat: 6g

Protein: 28g

# Copycat Taco Bell Crunch Wraps

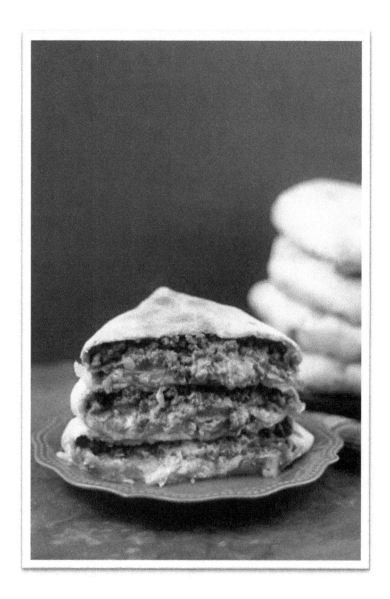

Preparation time: 15 minutes

Cooking time: 2 minutes

Servings: 6

**Ingredients:**

6 wheat tostadas

2 C. sour cream

2 C. Mexican blend cheese

2 C. shredded lettuce

12 ounces low-sodium nacho cheese

3 Roma tomatoes

6 12-inch wheat tortillas

1 1/3 C. water

2 packets low-sodium taco seasoning

2 pounds of lean ground beef

**Directions:**

Ensure your air fryer is preheated to 400 degrees. Make beef according to taco seasoning packets.

Place 2/3 cup prepared beef, 4 tbsp cheese, 1 tostada, 1/3 cup sour cream, 1/3 cup lettuce, 1/6 of tomatoes, and 1/3 cup cheese on each tortilla.

Fold up tortillas edges and repeat with remaining ingredients. Lay the folded sides of tortillas down into the air fryer and spray with olive oil.

Set temperature to 400°F, and set time to 2 minutes. Cook 2 minutes till browned.

**Nutrition:**

Calories: 530

Carbs: 71g

Fat: 21g

Protein: 16g

# Steak and Mushroom Gravy

Preparation time: 15 minutes

Cooking time: 15 minutes

Servings: 4

**Ingredients:**

4 cubed steaks

2 large eggs

1/2 dozen mushrooms

4 tablespoons unsalted butter

4 tablespoons black pepper

2 tablespoons salt

1/2 teaspoon onion powder

1/2 teaspoon garlic powder

1/4 teaspoon cayenne powder

1 1/4 teaspoons paprika

1 1/2 cups whole milk

1/3 cup flour

tablespoons vegetable oil

**Directions:**

Mix half of the flour and a pinch of black pepper in a shallow bowl or on a plate.

Beat 2 eggs in a bowl and mix in a pinch of salt and pepper.

Mix the other half of the flour with pepper to taste, garlic powder, paprika, cayenne, and onion powder in a separate shallow bowl.

Chop mushrooms and set aside.

Press your steak into the first flour mixture, then dip in egg, then press the steak into the second flour mixture until covered completely.

Set temperature to 360°F, and set time to 15 minutes, flipping halfway through.

While the steak cooks, warm the butter over medium heat and add mushrooms to sauté.

Add 4 tablespoons of the flour and pepper mix to the pan and mix until there are no clumps of flour.

Mix in whole milk and simmer. Serve over steak for breakfast, lunch, or dinner.

**Nutrition:**

Calories: 188

Carbs: 9g

Fat: 5g

Protein: 29g

# Chimichurri Skirt Steak

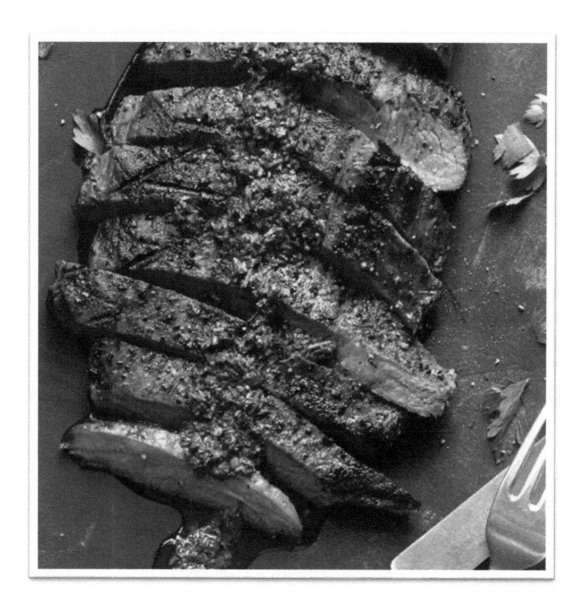

Preparation time: 10 minutes

Cooking time: 8 minutes

Servings: 2

**Ingredients:**

2 x 8 oz Skirt Steak

1 cup Finely Chopped Parsley

¼ cup Finely Chopped Mint

2 Tbsp Fresh Oregano (Washed & finely chopped)

3 Finely Chopped Cloves of Garlic

1 Tsp Red Pepper Flakes (Crushed)

1 Tbsp Ground Cumin

1 Tsp Cayenne Pepper

2 Tsp Smoked Paprika

1 Tsp Salt

¼ Tsp Pepper

¾ cup Oil

3 Tbsp Red Wine Vinegar

**Directions:**

Throw all the ingredients in a bowl (besides the steak) and mix well.

Put ¼ cup of the mixture in a plastic baggie with the steak and leave in the fridge overnight.

Leave the bag out at room temperature for at least 30 min before popping into the air fryer. Preheat for a minute or two to 390° F before cooking until med–rare (8–10 min).

Set temperature to 390°F, and set time to 10 minutes.

Put 2 Tbsp of the chimichurri mix on top of each steak before serving.

**Nutrition:**

Calories: 250

Carbs: 3g

Fat: 19g

Protein: 17g

# Country Fried Steak

Preparation time: 5 minutes

Cooking time: 12 minutes

Servings: 2

**Ingredients:**

1 tsp. pepper

2 C. almond milk

2 tbsp. almond flour

6 ounces ground sausage meat

1 tsp. pepper

1 tsp. salt

1 tsp. garlic powder

1 tsp. onion powder

1 C. panko breadcrumbs

1 C. almond flour

3 beaten eggs

6 ounces sirloin steak, pounded till thin

**Directions:**

Season panko breadcrumbs with spices. Dredge steak in flour, then egg, and then seasoned panko mixture.

Place into an air fryer basket. Set temperature to 370°F, and set time to 12 minutes.

To make sausage gravy, cook sausage and drain off fat, but reserve 2 tablespoons.

Add flour to sausage and mix until incorporated. Gradually mix in milk over medium to high heat until it becomes thick.

Season mixture with pepper and cook 3 minutes longer. Serve steak topped with gravy and enjoy.

**Nutrition:**

 Calories: 250

Carbs: 13g

Fat: 17g

Protein: 9g

# Creamy Burger & Potato Bake

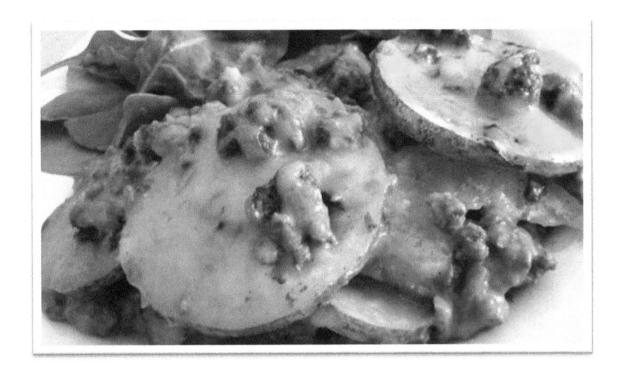

Preparation time: 5 minutes

Cooking time: 55 minutes

Servings: 3

**Ingredients:**

salt to taste

freshly ground pepper, to taste

1/2 (10.75 ounces) can condense cream of mushroom soup

1/2-pound lean ground beef

1-1/2 cups peeled and thinly sliced potatoes

1/2 cup shredded Cheddar cheese

1/4 cup chopped onion

1/4 cup and 2 tablespoons milk

**Directions:**

Lightly grease baking pan of the air fryer with cooking spray. Add ground beef. For 10 minutes, cook at 360°F. Stir and crumble halfway through cooking time.

Meanwhile, in a bowl, whisk well pepper, salt, milk, onion, and mushroom soup. Mix well.

Drain fat off ground beef and transfer beef to a plate.

In the same air fryer baking pan, layer ½ of potatoes on the bottom, then ½ of soup mixture, and then ½ of beef. Repeat process.

Cover pan with foil. Cook for 30 minutes. Remove the foil and cook again within 15 minutes or until potatoes are tender. Serve and enjoy.

**Nutrition:**

Calories: 103

Carbs: 4g

Fat: 9g

Protein: 2g

# Beefy 'n Cheesy Spanish Rice Casserole

Preparation time: 15 minutes

Cooking time: 50 minutes

Servings: 3

**Ingredients:**

2 tablespoons chopped green bell pepper

1 tablespoon chopped fresh cilantro

1/2-pound lean ground beef

1/2 cup water

1/2 teaspoon salt

1/2 teaspoon brown sugar

1/2 pinch ground black pepper

1/3 cup uncooked long-grain rice

1/4 cup finely chopped onion

1/4 cup Chile sauce

1/4 teaspoon ground cumin

1/4 teaspoon Worcestershire sauce

1/4 cup shredded Cheddar cheese

1/2 (14.5 ounces) can canned tomatoes

**Directions:**

Lightly grease baking pan of the air fryer with cooking spray. Add ground beef.

For 10 minutes, cook at 360°F. Halfway through cooking time, stir and crumble beef. Discard excess fat.

Stir in pepper, Worcestershire sauce, cumin, brown sugar, salt, Chile sauce, rice, water, tomatoes, green bell pepper, and onion.

Mix well. Cover the pan using a foil and cook for 25 minutes, stirring occasionally.

Give it one last good stir, press down firmly, and sprinkle cheese on top. Cook uncovered for 15 minutes at 390°F until tops are lightly browned. Serve and enjoy with chopped cilantro.

**Nutrition:**

Calories: 371

Carbs: 30g

Fat: 13g

Protein: 30g

# Warming Winter Beef with Celery

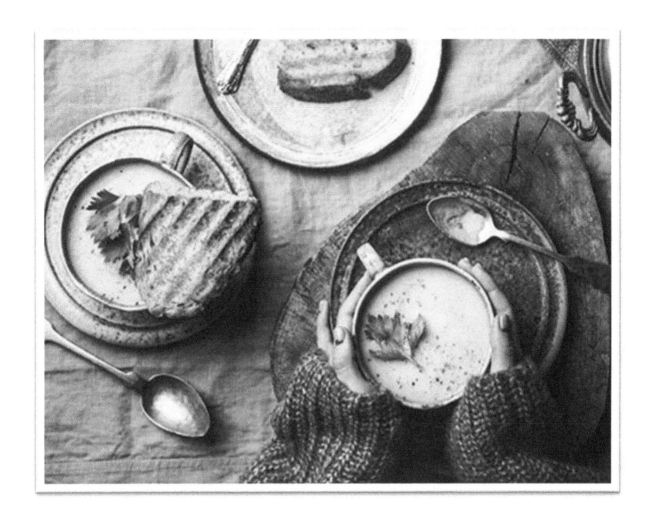

Preparation time: 5 minutes

Cooking time: 12 minutes

Servings: 4

**Ingredients:**

9 ounces tender beef, chopped

1/2 cup leeks, chopped

1/2 cup celery stalks, chopped

2 cloves garlic, smashed

2 tablespoons red cooking wine

3/4 cup cream of celery soup

2 sprigs rosemary, chopped

1/4 teaspoon smoked paprika

3/4 teaspoons salt

1/4 teaspoon black pepper

**Directions:**

Add the beef, leeks, celery, and garlic to the baking dish; cook for about 5 minutes at 390 degrees F.

Once the meat is starting to tender, pour in the wine and soup—season with rosemary, smoked paprika, salt, and black pepper. Now, cook an additional 7 minutes.

**Nutrition:**

Calories: 125

Carbs: 0g

Fat: 0g

Protein: 0g

# Beef & Veggie Spring Rolls

Preparation time: 15 minutes

Cooking time: 12 minutes

Servings: 10

**Ingredients:**

2-ounce Asian rice noodles

1 tablespoon sesame oil

7-ounce ground beef

1 small onion, chopped

3 garlic cloves, crushed

1 cup of fresh mixed vegetables

1 teaspoon soy sauce

1 packet spring roll skins

2 tablespoons water

Olive oil, as required

**Directions:**

Dip the noodles in warm water until soft.

Drain and cut into small lengths. Heat the oil in a pan and add the onion and garlic and sauté for about 4-5 minutes.

Add beef and cook for about 4-5 minutes. Add vegetables and cook for about 5-7 minutes or till cooked through.

Stir in soy sauce and remove from the heat. Stir in the noodles and keep aside till all the juices have been absorbed.

Preheat the air fryer oven to 350 degrees F. Place the spring rolls skin onto a smooth surface.

Add a line of the filling diagonally across. Fold the top point over the filling and then fold in both sides.

On the final point, brush it with water before rolling to seal. Brush the spring rolls with oil.

Arrange the rolls in batches in the air fryer and Cook for about 8 minutes. Repeat with remaining rolls. Now, place spring rolls onto a baking sheet — Bake for about 6 minutes per side.

**Nutrition:**

Calories: 160

Carbs: 0g

Fat: 0g

Protein: 7g

# Charred Onions and Steak Cube BBQ

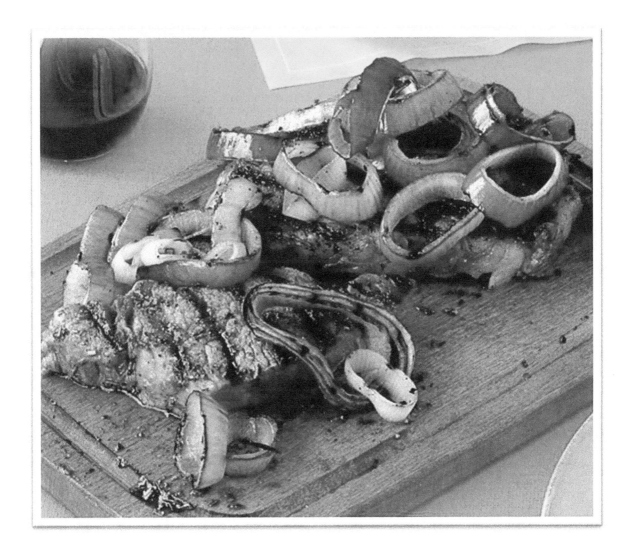

Preparation time: 5 minutes

Cooking time: 40 minutes

Servings: 3

**Ingredients:**

1 cup red onions, cut into wedges

1 tablespoon dry mustard

1 tablespoon olive oil

1-pound boneless beef sirloin, cut into cubes

Salt and pepper to taste

**Directions:**

Preheat the air fryer to 390°F. Place the grill pan accessory in the air fryer.

Toss all the fixings in a bowl and mix until everything is coated with the seasonings.

Put on the grill pan and cook for 40 minutes. Halfway through the cooking time, give a stir to cook evenly.

**Nutrition:**

Calories: 120

Carbs: 0g

Fat: 0g

Protein: 18g

# Beef Stroganoff

Preparation time: 15 minutes

Cooking time: 14 minutes

Servings: 4

**Ingredients:**

9 oz. Tender Beef

1 Onion, chopped

1 Tbsp Paprika

3/4 Cup Sour Cream

Salt and pepper to taste

Baking Dish

**Directions:**

Preheat the air fryer oven to 390 degrees. Slice the beef, then marinate it with the paprika.

Add the chopped onions into the baking dish and heat for about 2 minutes in the air fryer oven.

When the onions are transparent, add the beef into the dish and cook for 5 minutes.

Once the beef is starting to tender, pour in the sour cream and cook for another 7 minutes.

Season with salt and pepper and serve.

**Nutrition:**

Calories: 127

Carbs: 9g

Fat: 9g

Protein: 6g

# Cheesy Ground Beef and Mac Taco Casserole

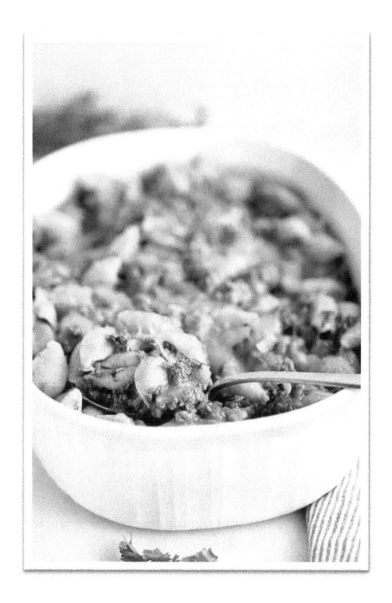

Preparation time: 15 minutes

Cooking time: 25 minutes

Servings: 5

## Ingredients:

1-ounce shredded Cheddar cheese

1-ounce shredded Monterey Jack cheese

2 tablespoons chopped green onions

1/2 (10.75 ounces) can condensed tomato soup

1/2-pound lean ground beef

1/2 cup crushed tortilla chips

1/4-pound macaroni, cooked according to manufacturer's Instructions

1/4 cup chopped onion

1/4 cup sour cream (optional)

1/2 (1.25 ounce) package taco seasoning mix

1/2 can diced tomatoes

## Directions:

Lightly grease baking pan of the air fryer with cooking spray. Add onion and ground beef. For 10 minutes, cook at 360°F. Halfway through cooking time, stir and crumble ground beef.

Add taco seasoning, diced tomatoes, and tomato soup. Mix well. Mix in pasta.

Sprinkle crushed tortilla chips. Sprinkle cheese.

Cook for 15 minutes at 390°F until tops are lightly browned, and cheese is melted.

Serve and enjoy.

**Nutrition:**

Calories: 225

Carbs: 16g

Fat: 8g

Protein: 25g

# Ham and Cheese Rollups

Preparation time: 5 minutes

Cooking time: 8 minutes

Servings: 12

**Ingredients:**

2 tsp. raw honey

2 tsp. dried parsley

1 tbsp. poppy seeds

½ C. melted coconut oil

¼ C. spicy brown mustard

9 slices of provolone cheese

10 ounces of thinly sliced Black Forest Ham

1 tube of crescent rolls

**Directions:**

Roll out dough into a rectangle. Spread 2-3 tablespoons of spicy mustard onto the dough, then layer provolone cheese and ham slices. Roll the filled dough up as tight as you can and slice into 12-15 pieces.

Melt coconut oil and mix with a pinch of salt and pepper, parsley, honey, and the rest of the mustard.

Brush mustard mixture over roll-ups and sprinkle with poppy seeds. Grease the air fryer oven basket liberally with olive oil and add roll-ups.

Set oven to Air Fry at 350°F, and set time to 8 minutes. Serve.

**Nutrition:**

Calories: 280

Carbs: 27g

Fat: 13g

Protein: 13g

# Pork Taquitos

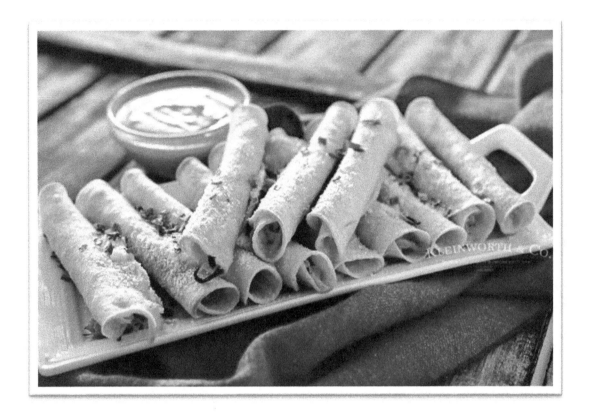

Preparation time: 15 minutes

Cooking time: 16 minutes

Servings: 8

**Ingredients:**

1 juiced lime

10 whole-wheat tortillas

2 ½ C. shredded mozzarella cheese

30 ounces of cooked and shredded pork tenderloin

**Directions:**

Ensure your air fryer oven is preheated to 380 degrees. Drizzle pork with lime juice and gently mix.

Warm the tortillas in the microwave with a dampened paper towel to soften. Add about 3 ounces of pork and ¼ cup of shredded cheese to each tortilla.

Tightly roll them up. Spray the air fryer oven basket with a bit of olive oil.

Set oven to Air Fry at 380°F, and set time to 10 minutes. Air fry taquitos 7-10 minutes till tortillas turn a slight golden color, making sure to flip halfway through the cooking process.

**Nutrition:**

Calories: 210

Carbs: 25g

Fat: 9g

Protein: 7g

# Juicy Pork Ribs Ole

Preparation time: 15 minutes

Cooking time: 25 minutes

Servings: 4

**Ingredients:**

1 rack of pork ribs

1/2 cup low-fat milk

1 tablespoon taco seasoning mix

1 can tomato sauce

1/2 teaspoon ground black pepper

1 teaspoon seasoned salt

1 tablespoon cornstarch

1 teaspoon canola oil

**Directions:**

Place all ingredients in a mixing dish; let them marinate for 1 hour.

Cook the marinated ribs approximately 25 minutes at 390 degrees F. Work with batches.

Enjoy

**Nutrition:**

Calories: 240

Carbs: 0g

Fat: 17g

Protein: 54g

# Pork Tenders with Bell Peppers

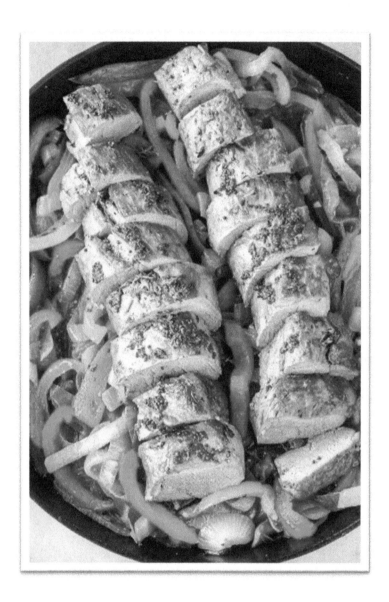

Preparation time: 15 minutes

Cooking time: 15 minutes

Servings: 4

**Ingredients:**

11 oz Pork Tenderloin

1 Bell Pepper, in thin strips

1 Red Onion, sliced

2 tsp. Provencal Herbs

Black Pepper to taste

1 tbsp Olive Oil

1/2 tbsp Mustard

**Directions:**

Preheat the Air fryer oven to 390 degrees.

In the oven dish, mix the bell pepper strips with the onion, herbs, and salt plus pepper to taste.

Put half a tablespoon of olive oil to the batter.

Slice the pork tenderloin into four pieces and rub with salt, pepper, and mustard.

Thinly coat the pieces with remaining olive oil and place them upright in the oven pan on top of the pepper mixture.

Set it to 15 minutes, then roast the meat and the vegetables. Turn the pork meat and mix the peppers halfway through. Serve with a fresh salad.

**Nutrition:**

Calories: 310

Carbs: 30g

Fat: 9g

Protein: 28g

# Cajun Bacon Pork Loin Fillet

Preparation time: 1 hour & 15 minutes

Cooking time: 20 minutes

Servings: 6

**Ingredients:**

1½ pounds pork loin fillet or pork tenderloin

3 tablespoons olive oil

2 tablespoons Cajun Spice Mix

Salt

6 slices bacon

Olive oil spray

**Directions:**

Slice the pork in half so that it will fit in the air fryer basket.

Place both pieces of meat in a resealable plastic bag. Add the oil, Cajun seasoning, and salt to taste, if using.

Seal the bag and massage to coat all of the meat with the oil and seasonings. Marinate in the fridge within 1 hour or up to 24 hours.

Remove the pork from the bag and wrap 3 bacon slices around each piece. Spray the Air Fryer Oven basket with olive oil spray. Place the meat in the Air Fryer Oven basket.

Set oven to Air Fry at 350°F for 15 minutes. Increase the temperature to 400°F for 5 minutes. Use a meat thermometer to ensure the meat has reached an internal temperature of 145°F.

Let the meat rest for 10 minutes. Slice into 6 medallions and serve.

**Nutrition:**

Calories: 190

Carbs: 5g

Fat: 9g

Protein: 23g

# Scotch Eggs

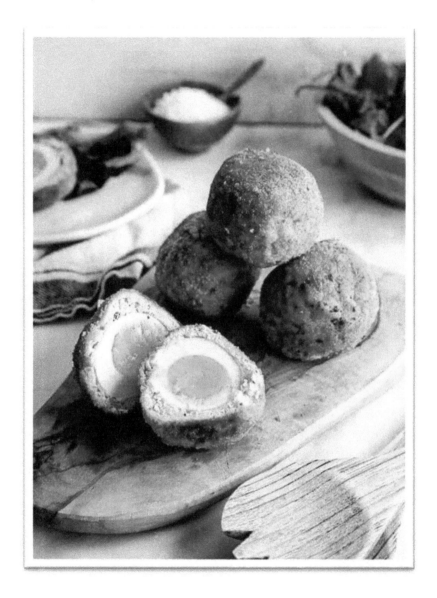

Preparation time: 15 minutes

Cooking time: 15 minutes

Servings: 8

## Ingredients:

2 pounds ground pork or ground beef

2 teaspoons sea salt

½ teaspoon ground black pepper

8 large hard-boiled eggs, peeled

2 cups of pork dust

Dijon mustard, for serving (optional)

## Directions:

Spray the Air Fryer Oven basket using the avocado oil. Preheat the air fryer oven to 400°F.

Put the ground pork in a bowl, put the salt and pepper, and use your hands to mix until seasoned throughout.

Flatten about ¼ pound of ground pork in the palm of your hand and place a peeled egg in the center. Fold the pork entirely around the egg.

Repeat with the remaining eggs. Place the pork dust in a medium-sized bowl.

One at a time, roll the ground pork–covered eggs in the pork dust and use your hands to press it into the eggs to form a nice crust.

Place the eggs in the Air Fryer Oven basket and spray them with avocado oil.

Set oven to Air Fry at 400°F. Cook the eggs for 15 minutes, or until the pork's internal temperature reaches 145°F and the outside is golden brown.

Garnish with ground black pepper and serve with Dijon mustard, if desired.

## Nutrition:

Calories: 306

Carbs: 20g

Fat: 19g

Protein: 12g

# Asian Pork Chops

Preparation time: 2 hours & 15 minutes

Cooking time: 15 minutes

Servings: 4

**Ingredients:**

1/2 cup hoisin sauce

3 tablespoons cider vinegar

1 tablespoon Asian sweet chili sauce

1/4 teaspoon garlic powder

4 (1/2-inch-thick) boneless pork chops

1 teaspoon salt

1/2 teaspoon pepper

**Directions:**

Stir hoisin, chili sauce, garlic powder, plus vinegar in a mixing bowl.

Separate 1/4 cup of this batter, add pork chops to the bowl and marinate in the fridge for 2 hours. Remove the pork chops and place them on a plate.

Sprinkle each side of the pork chop evenly with salt and pepper.

Cook at 360 degrees for 14 minutes, flipping halfway through.

**Nutrition:**

Calories: 359

Carbs: 5g

Fat: 8g

Protein: 50g

# BBQ Riblets

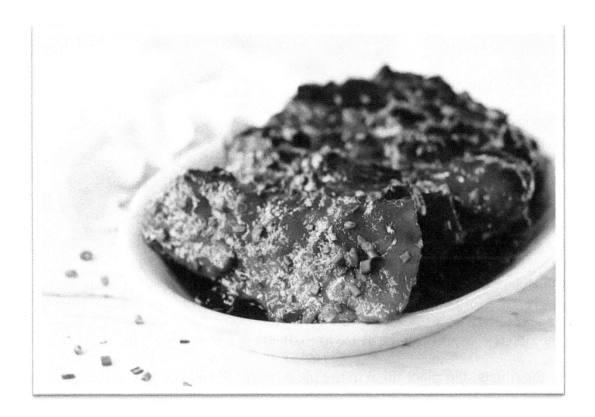

Preparation time: 15 minutes

Cooking time: 25 minutes

Servings: 4

**Ingredients:**

1 rack pork riblets, cut into individual riblets

1 teaspoon fine sea salt

1 teaspoon ground black pepper

Sauce:

¼ cup apple cider vinegar

¼ cup beef broth

¼ cup Swerve confectioners'-style sweetener or powdered sweetener

¼ cup tomato sauce

1 teaspoon liquid smoke

1 teaspoon onion powder

2 cloves garlic, minced

**Directions:**

Spray the Air Fryer Oven basket with avocado oil. Preheat the air fryer oven to 350°F. Season the riblets well on all sides with the salt and pepper.

Place the riblets in the air fryer basket, then onto the Baking Pan. Set oven to Air Fry at 350°F, and cook for 10 minutes, flipping halfway through.

While the riblets cook, mix all the sauce ingredients in a 6-inch pie pan.

Remove the riblets, and place them in the pie pan with the sauce. Stir to coat the riblets in the sauce.

Transfer the pan to the Air Fryer Oven and cook for 10 to 15 minutes, until the pork is cooked through and the internal temperature reaches 145°F. Serve.

**Nutrition:**

Calories: 220

Carbs: 35g

Fat: 4g

Protein: 18g

# Bacon-Wrapped Stuffed Pork Chops

Preparation time: 15 minutes

Cooking time: 20 minutes

Servings: 4

**Ingredients:**

4 (1-inch-thick) boneless pork chops

2 (5.2-ounce) packages Boursin cheese

8 slices thin-cut bacon

**Directions:**

Grease the Air Fryer Oven basket with avocado oil. Preheat the air fryer oven to 400°F.

Place one of the chops on a cutting board. Make a 1-inch-wide incision on the top edge of the chop.

Carefully cut into the chop to form a large pocket, leaving a ½-inch border along the sides and bottom. Repeat with the other 3 chops. Snip the corner of a large resealable plastic bag to form a ¾-inch hole.

Place the Boursin cheese in the bag and pipe the cheese into the pockets in the chops, dividing the cheese evenly among them.

Wrap 2 slices of bacon around each chop and secure the ends with toothpicks.

Place the bacon-wrapped chops in the Air Fryer Oven basket. Set oven to Air Fry at 400°F and cook for 10 minutes, then flip the chops and cook for another 8 to 10 minutes, until the bacon is crisp, the chops are cooked through, and the internal temperature reaches 145°F.

**Nutrition:**

Calories: 150

Carbs: 1g

Fat: 6g

Protein: 22g

# Panko-Breaded Pork Chops

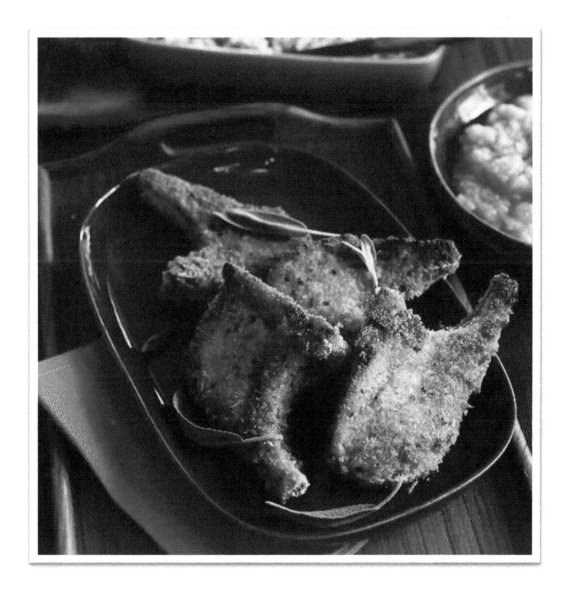

Preparation time: 15 minutes

Cooking time: 12 minutes

Servings: 6

**Ingredients:**

5 (3½- to 5-ounce) pork chops

Seasoning salt

Pepper

¼ cup all-purpose flour

2 tablespoons panko bread crumbs

Cooking oil

**Directions:**

Rub the pork chops using a salt and pepper to taste.

Put the flour on both sides of the pork chops, then coat both sides with panko bread crumbs.

Put the pork chops in the air fryer basket. Stacking them is okay.

Spray the pork chops with cooking oil. Set oven to Air Fry at 400°F. Cook for 6 minutes.

Flip the pork chops. Cook for an additional 6 minutes. Cool before serving.

**Nutrition:**

Calories: 253

Carbs: 7g

Fat: 14g

Protein: 26g

# Cajun Pork Steaks

Preparation time: 15 minutes

Cooking time: 20 minutes

Servings: 6

**Ingredients:**

4-6 pork steaks

BBQ sauce:

Cajun seasoning

1 tbsp. vinegar

1 tsp. low-sodium soy sauce

½ C. brown sugar

½ C. vegan ketchup

**Directions:**

Ensure your air fryer oven is preheated to 290 degrees. Sprinkle pork steaks with Cajun seasoning.

Combine remaining ingredients and brush onto steaks. Add coated steaks to Air Fryer Oven basket.

Set oven to "Air Fry" at 290°F, and set time to 20 minutes. Cook 15-20 minutes till just browned.

**Nutrition:**

Calories: 229

Carbs: 2g

Fat: 10g

Protein: 32g

# Porchetta-Style Pork Chops

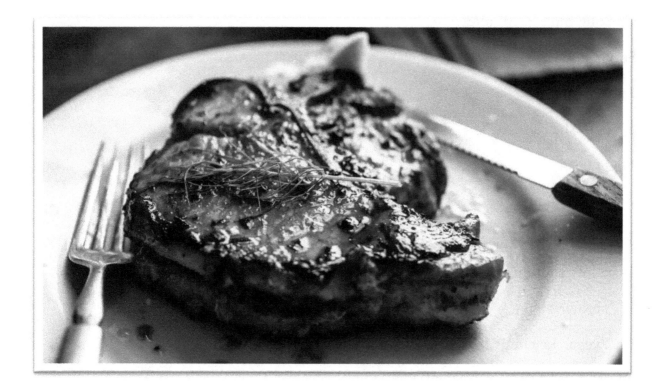

Preparation time: 15 minutes

Cooking time: 15 minutes

Servings: 2

**Ingredients:**

1 tablespoon extra-virgin olive oil

Grated zest of 1 lemon

2 cloves garlic, minced

2 teaspoons chopped fresh rosemary

1 teaspoon finely chopped fresh sage

1 teaspoon fennel seeds, lightly crushed

¼ to ½ teaspoon red pepper flakes

1 teaspoon kosher salt

1 teaspoon black pepper

(8-ounce) center-cut bone-in pork chops, about 1 inch thick

**Directions:**

In a small bowl, combine the olive oil, zest, garlic, rosemary, sage, fennel seeds, red pepper, salt, and black pepper.

Stir, crushing the herbs with the back of a spoon, until a paste form. Rub the seasoning mix on each side of the pork chops.

Put the chops inside the air fryer basket—set oven to "Air Fry" at 375°F for 15 minutes. Serve.

**Nutrition:**

Calories: 250

Carbs: 15g

Fat: 9g

Protein: 34g

# Dry Rub Baby Back Ribs

Preparation time: 15 minutes

Cooking time: 35 minutes

Servings: 2

**Ingredients:**

2 teaspoons fine sea salt

1 teaspoon ground black pepper

2 teaspoons smoked paprika

1 teaspoon garlic powder

1 teaspoon onion powder

½ teaspoon chili powder (optional)

1 rack baby back ribs, half crosswise

**Directions:**

Grease your Air Fryer Oven basket with avocado oil. Preheat the air fryer oven to 350°F. Mix the salt, pepper, and seasonings in a small bowl. Season the ribs on all sides with the seasoning mixture.

Place the ribs in the air fryer basket, then set oven to Air Fry at 350°F, cook for 15 minutes, then flip the ribs over and cook for another 15 to 20 minutes.

**Nutrition:**

Calories: 64

Carbs: 15g

Fat: 1g

Protein: 1g

# Pork Milanese

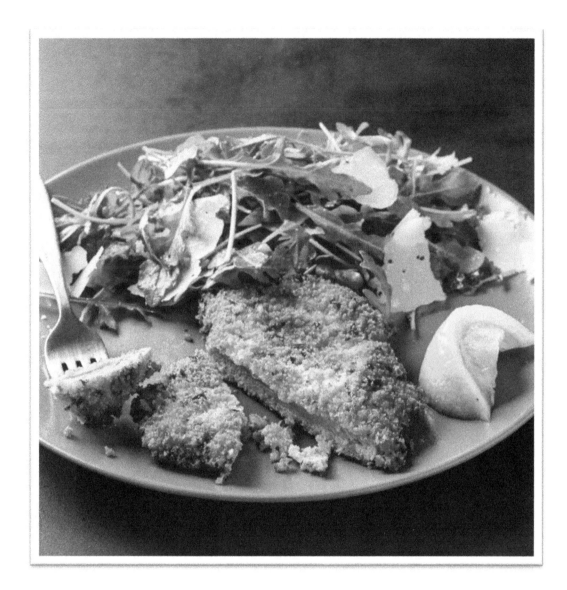

Preparation time: 15 minutes

Cooking time: 12 minutes

Servings: 4

**Ingredients:**

4 (1-inch) boneless pork chops

Fine sea salt and ground black pepper

2 large eggs

¾ cup powdered Parmesan cheese about 2¼ ounces

Chopped fresh parsley, for garnish

Lemon slices, for serving

**Directions:**

Spray the air fryer basket using avocado oil. Preheat the air fryer oven to 400°F.

Put the pork chops in the middle of 2 sheets of plastic wrap and pound them with the flat side of a meat tenderizer until they're ¼ inch thick.

Lightly season both sides of the chops with salt and pepper. Lightly beat the eggs in a shallow bowl.

Divide the Parmesan cheese evenly between 2 bowls and set the bowls in this order: Parmesan, eggs, Parmesan.

Dredge a chop in the first bowl of Parmesan, then dip it in the eggs, and then dredge it again in the second bowl of Parmesan, making sure both sides and all edges are well coated. Repeat with the remaining chops.

Place the chops in the Air Fryer Oven basket and cook for 12 minutes, or until the internal temperature reaches 145°F, flipping halfway through.

Garnish with fresh parsley, then serve with lemon slices.

**Nutrition:**

Calories: 200

Carbs: 15g

Fat: 5g

Protein: 21g

# Roasted Pork Tenderloin

Preparation time: 15 minutes

Cooking time: 1 hour

Servings: 4

**Ingredients:**

1 (3-pound) pork tenderloin

2 tablespoons extra-virgin olive oil

2 garlic cloves, minced

1 teaspoon dried basil

1 teaspoon dried oregano

1 teaspoon dried thyme

Salt

Pepper

**Directions:**

Greased the pork tenderloin with the olive oil. Massage the garlic, basil, oregano, thyme, and salt and pepper to taste all over the tenderloin.

Place the tenderloin in the Air fryer basket. Set oven to "Air Fry" at 400°F. Cook for 45 minutes. Use a meat thermometer to test for doneness.

Open the oven and flip the pork tenderloin—Cook for an additional 15 minutes. Remove the cooked pork from the Air Fryer Oven and allow it to rest for 10 minutes before cutting.

**Nutrition:**

Calories: 46

Carbs: 0g

Fat: 1g

Protein: 8g

# Juicy Pork Chops

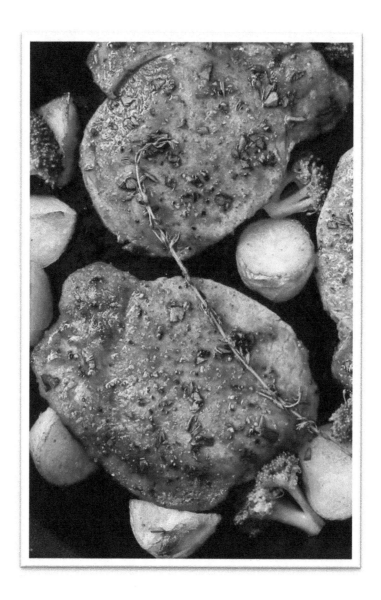

Preparation Time: 10 minutes

Cooking Time: 16 minutes

Servings: 4

**Ingredients:**

4 pork chops, boneless

2 tsp olive oil

½ tsp celery seed

½ tsp parsley

½ tsp granulated onion

½ tsp granulated garlic

¼ tsp sugar

½ tsp salt

**Directions:**

In a small bowl, mix oil, celery seed, parsley, granulated onion, granulated garlic, sugar, and salt.

Rub seasoning mixture all over the pork chops.

Place pork chops on the air fryer oven pan and cook at 350 F for 8 minutes.

Turn pork chops on its other side and cook for 8 minutes more.

Serve and enjoy.

**Nutrition:**

Calories 279

Fat 22.3 g

Carbohydrates 0.6 g

Sugar 0.3 g

Protein 18.1 g

Cholesterol 69 mg

# Crispy Meatballs

Preparation Time: 10 minutes

Cooking Time: 12 minutes

Servings: 8

**Ingredients:**

1 lb. ground pork

1 lb. ground beef

1 tbsp Worcestershire sauce

½ cup feta cheese, crumbled

½ cup breadcrumbs

2 eggs, lightly beaten

¼ cup fresh parsley, chopped

1 tbsp garlic, minced

1 onion, chopped

¼ tsp pepper

1 tsp salt

**Directions:**

Put all the fixings into the mixing bowl and mix until well combined.

Spray the tray pan with cooking spray.

Make small balls from meat mixture and arrange on a pan and air fry t 400 F for 10-12 minutes.

Serve and enjoy.

**Nutrition:**

Calories 263

Fat 9 g

Carbohydrates 7.5 g

Sugar 1.9 g

Protein 35.9 g

Cholesterol 141 mg

# Flavourful Steak

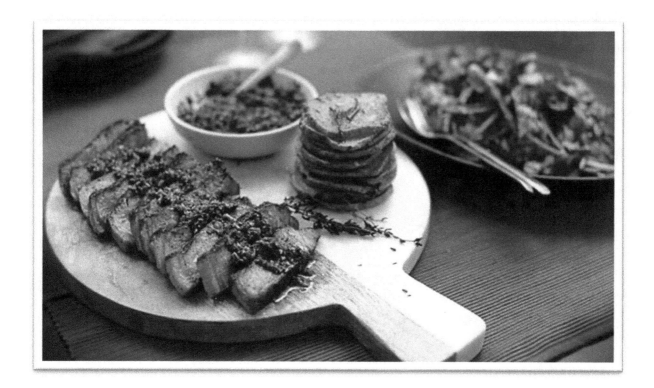

Preparation Time: 10 minutes

Cooking Time: 18 minutes

Servings: 2

**Ingredients:**

2 steaks, rinsed and pat dry

½ tsp garlic powder

1 tsp olive oil

Pepper

Salt

**Directions:**

Massage the steaks with olive oil and season with garlic powder, pepper, and salt.

Preheat the air fryer oven to 400 F.

Place steaks on air fryer oven pan and air fry for 10-18 minutes. Turn halfway through.

Serve and enjoy.

**Nutrition:**

Calories 361

Fat 10.9 g

Carbohydrates 0.5 g

Sugar 0.2 g

Protein 61.6 g

Cholesterol 153 mg

# Lemon Garlic Lamb Chops

Preparation Time: 10 minutes

Cooking Time: 6 minutes

Servings: 6

**Ingredients:**

6 lamb loin chops

2 tbsp fresh lemon juice

1 ½ tbsp lemon zest

1 tbsp dried rosemary

1 tbsp olive oil

1 tbsp garlic, minced

Pepper

Salt

**Directions:**

Add lamb chops in a mixing bowl.

Add remaining ingredients on top of lamb chops and coat well.

Arrange the meat lambs on the air fryer oven tray and air fry at 400 F within 3 minutes.

Turn lamb chops to another side and air fry for 3 minutes more.

Serve and enjoy.

**Nutrition:**

Calories 69

Fat 6 g

Carbohydrates 1.2 g

Sugar 0.2 g

Protein 3 g

Cholesterol 0 mg

# Honey Mustard Pork Tenderloin

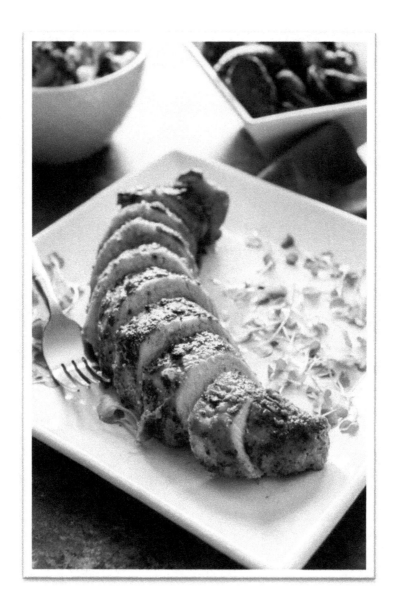

Preparation Time: 10 minutes

Cooking Time: 26 minutes

Servings: 4

## Ingredients:

1 lb. pork tenderloin

1 tsp sriracha sauce

1 tbsp garlic, minced

2 tbsp soy sauce

1 ½ tbsp honey

¾ tbsp Dijon mustard

1 tbsp mustard

## Directions:

Add sriracha sauce, garlic, soy sauce, honey, Dijon mustard, and mustard into the large zip-lock bag and mix well.

Add pork tenderloin into the bag. Seal, then place it in the refrigerator overnight.

Preheat the air fryer oven to 380 F.

Spray the air fryer tray with cooking spray, then place marinated pork tenderloin on a tray and air fry for 26 minutes. Turn pork tenderloin after every 5 minutes.

Slice and serve.

## Nutrition:

Calories 195

Fat 4.1 g

Carbohydrates 8 g

Sugar 6.7 g

Protein 30.5 g

Cholesterol 83 mg

# Easy Rosemary Lamb Chops

Preparation Time: 10 minutes

Cooking Time: 6 minutes

Servings: 4

**Ingredients:**

4 lamb chops

2 tbsp dried rosemary

¼ cup fresh lemon juice

Pepper

Salt

**Directions:**

In a small bowl, mix lemon juice, rosemary, pepper, and salt.

Brush the lemon juice rosemary mixture over lamb chops.

Place lamb chops on air fryer oven tray and air fry setting at 400 F for 3 minutes.

Turn lamb chops to the other side and cook for 3 minutes more.

Serve and enjoy.

**Nutrition:**

Calories 267

Fat 21.7 g

Carbohydrates 1.4 g

Sugar 0.3 g

Protein 16.9 g

# Juicy Steak Bites

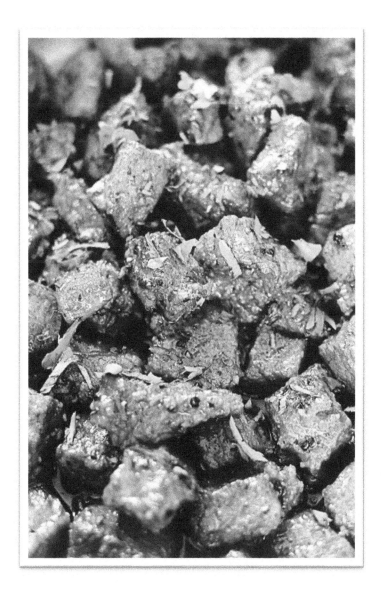

Preparation Time: 10 minutes

Cooking Time: 9 minutes

Servings: 4

## Ingredients:

1 lb. sirloin steak, cut into bite-size pieces

1 tbsp steak seasoning

1 tbsp olive oil

Pepper

Salt

## Directions:

Preheat the air fryer oven to 390 F.

Add steak pieces into the large mixing bowl. Add steak seasoning, oil, pepper, and salt over steak pieces and toss until well coated.

Transfer steak pieces to air fryer pan and air fry for 5 minutes.

Turn the steak pieces to the other side and cook for 4 minutes more. Serve and enjoy.

## Nutrition:

Calories 241

Fat 10.6 g

Carbohydrates 0 g

Sugar 0 g

Protein 34.4 g

Cholesterol 101 mg

# Greek Lamb Chops

Preparation Time: 10 minutes

Cooking Time: 10 minutes

Servings: 4

**Ingredients:**

2 lbs. lamb chops

2 tsp garlic, minced

1 ½ tsp dried oregano

¼ cup fresh lemon juice

¼ cup olive oil

½ tsp pepper

1 tsp salt

**Directions:**

Add lamb chops in a mixing bowl. Add remaining ingredients over the lamb chops and coat well.

Arrange lamb chops on the air fryer oven tray and cook at 400 F for 5 minutes.

Turn lamb chops and cook for 5 minutes more.

Serve and enjoy.

**Nutrition:**

Calories 538

Fat 29.4 g

Carbohydrates 1.3 g

Sugar 0.4 g

Protein 64 g

Cholesterol 204 mg

# Easy Beef Roast

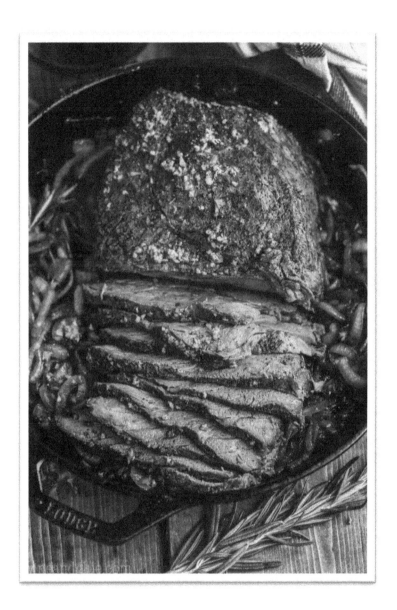

Preparation Time: 10 minutes

Cooking Time: 45 minutes

Servings: 6

**Ingredients:**

2 ½ lbs. beef roast

2 tbsp Italian seasoning

**Directions:**

Arrange roast on the rotisserie spite.

Rub roast with Italian seasoning then insert into the air fryer oven.

Air fry at 350 F for 45 minutes or until the roast's internal temperature reaches 145 F.

Slice and serve.

**Nutrition:**

Calories 365

Fat 13.2 g

Carbohydrates 0.5 g

Sugar 0.4 g

Protein 57.4 g

Cholesterol 172 mg

# Herb Butter Rib-eye Steak

Preparation Time: 10 minutes

Cooking Time: 14 minutes

Servings: 4

**Ingredients:**

2 lb. rib eye steak, bone-in

1 tsp fresh rosemary, chopped

1 tsp fresh thyme, chopped

1 tsp fresh chives, chopped

2 tsp fresh parsley, chopped

1 tsp garlic, minced

¼ cup butter softened

Pepper

Salt

**Directions:**

Mix the butter plus herbs in a small bowl.

Rub herb butter on rib-eye steak and place it in the refrigerator for 30 minutes.

Place marinated steak on air fryer oven pan and cook at 400 F for 12-14 minutes.

Serve and enjoy.

**Nutrition:**

Calories 416

Fat 36.7 g

Carbohydrates 0.7 g

Sugar 0 g

Protein 20.3 g

Cholesterol 106 mg

# BBQ Pork Chops

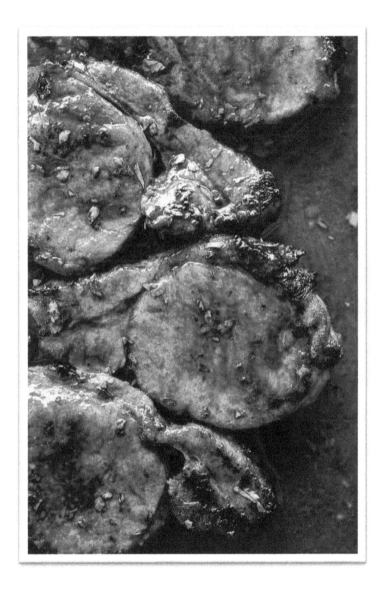

Preparation Time: 10 minutes

Cooking Time: 7 minutes

Servings: 4

## Ingredients:

4 pork chops

For rub:

½ tsp allspice

½ tsp dry mustard

1 tsp ground cumin

1 tsp garlic powder

½ tsp chili powder

½ tsp paprika

1 tbsp brown sugar

1 tsp salt

## Directions:

Mix all the rub fixings in a small bowl and rub all over pork chops.

Arrange pork chops on air fryer tray and air fry at 400 F for 5.

Turn pork chops on its other side and air fry for 2 minutes more.

Serve and enjoy.

## Nutrition:

Calories 273

Fat 20.2 g

Carbohydrates 3.4 g

Sugar 2.4 g

Protein 18.4 g

Cholesterol 69 mg

# Simple Beef Patties

Preparation Time: 10 minutes

Cooking Time: 13 minutes

Servings: 4

**Ingredients:**

1 lb. ground beef

½ tsp garlic powder

¼ tsp onion powder

Pepper

Salt

**Directions:**

Preheat the air fryer oven to 400 F.

Add ground meat, garlic powder, onion powder, pepper, and salt into the mixing bowl and mix until well combined.

Make even shape patties from meat mixture and arrange at air fryer pan.

Cook patties for 10 minutes. Turn patties after 5 minutes. Serve and enjoy.

**Nutrition:**

Calories 212

Fat 7.1 g

Carbohydrates 0.4 g

Sugar 0.1 g

Protein 34.5 g

Cholesterol 101 mg

# Marinated Pork Chops

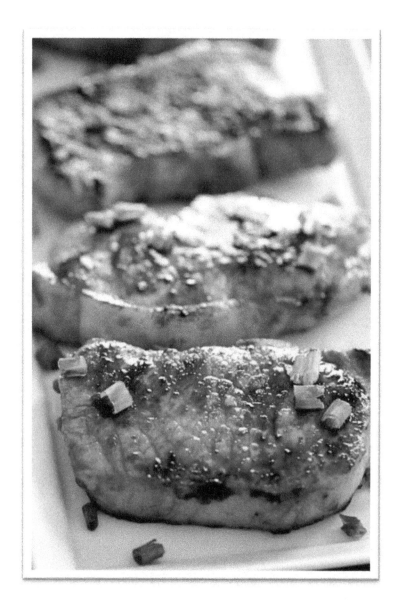

Preparation Time: 10 minutes

Cooking Time: 30 minutes

Servings: 2

**Ingredients:**

2 pork chops, boneless

1 tsp garlic powder

½ cup flour

1 cup buttermilk

Pepper

Salt

**Directions:**

Add pork chops and buttermilk in a zip-lock bag. Seal the bag and place it properly in the refrigerator overnight.

In another zip-lock bag, add flour, garlic powder, pepper, and salt.

Remove marinated pork chops from buttermilk and add in flour mixture and shake until well coated.

Preheat the air fryer oven to 380 F.

Grease air fryer tray with cooking spray.

Arrange pork chops on a tray and air fryer for 28-30 minutes.

Turn pork chops after 18 minutes. Serve and enjoy.

**Nutrition:**

Calories 424

Fat 21.3 g

Carbohydrates 30.8 g

Sugar 6.3 g

Protein 25.5 g

Cholesterol 74 mg

# Pork Satay

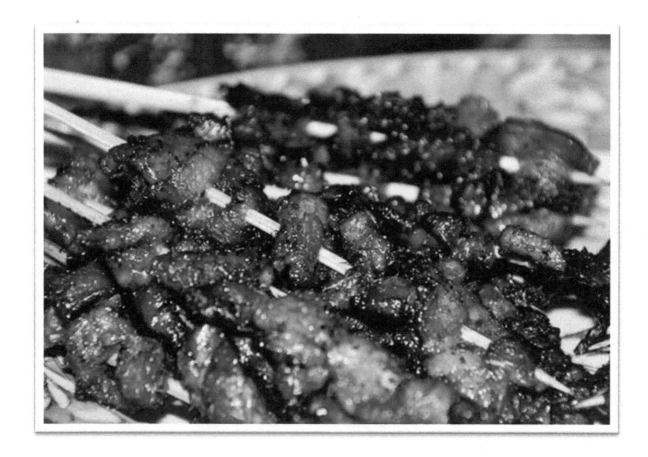

Preparation time: 15 minutes

Cooking time: 14 minutes

Servings: 4

**Ingredients:**

1 (1-pound) pork tenderloin, cut into 1½-inch cubes

¼ cup minced onion

2 garlic cloves, minced

1 jalapeño pepper, minced

2 tablespoons freshly squeezed lime juice

2 tablespoons coconut milk

2 tablespoons unsalted peanut butter

2 teaspoons curry powder

**Directions:**

In a medium bowl, mix the pork, onion, garlic, jalapeño, lime juice, coconut milk, peanut butter, and curry powder until well combined. Set aside within 10 minutes at room temperature.

With a slotted spoon, remove the pork from the marinade. Reserve the marinade.

Thread the pork onto about 8 bamboo or metal skewers. Grill for 9 to 14 minutes, brushing once with the reserved marinade until the pork reaches at least 145°F on a meat thermometer.

Discard any remaining marinade. Serve immediately.

**Nutrition:**

Calories: 194

Fat: 7g

Protein: 25g

Carbohydrates: 7g

Sodium: 65mg

Fiber: 1g

Sugar: 3g

# Pork Burgers with Red Cabbage Salad

Preparation time: 15 minutes

Cooking time: 9 minutes

Servings: 4

**Ingredients:**

½ cup Greek yogurt

2 tablespoons low-sodium mustard, divided

1 tablespoon lemon juice

¼ cup sliced red cabbage

¼ cup grated carrots

1-pound lean ground pork

½ teaspoon paprika

1 cup mixed baby lettuce greens

2 small tomatoes, sliced

8 small low-sodium whole-wheat sandwich buns, cut in half

**Directions:**

In a small bowl, combine the yogurt, 1 tablespoon mustard, lemon juice, cabbage, and carrots; mix and refrigerate.

In a medium bowl, combine the pork, remaining 1 tablespoon mustard, and paprika. Form into 8 small patties.

Put the sliders into the air fryer basket. Grill for 7 to 9 minutes, or until the sliders register 165°F as tested with a meat thermometer.

Assemble the burgers by placing some of the lettuce greens on a bun bottom. Top with a tomato slice, the -burgers, and the cabbage mixture. Add the bun top and serve immediately.

**Nutrition:**

Calories: 472

Fat 15g

Protein: 35g

Carbohydrates: 51g

Sodium 138mg

Sugar 8g

Fiber 8g

# Crispy Mustard Pork Tenderloin

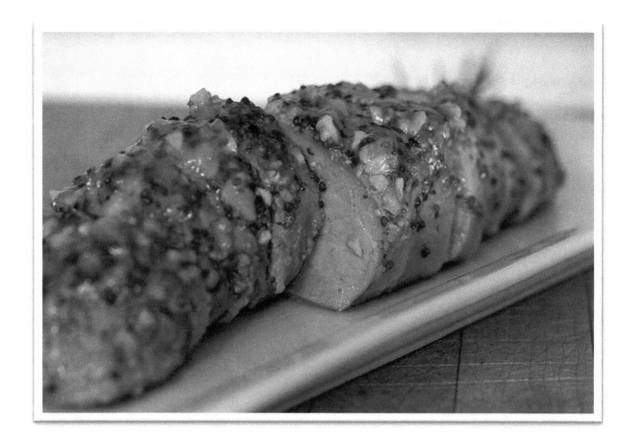

Preparation time: 15 minutes

Cooking time: 16 minutes

Servings: 4

**Ingredients:**

3 tablespoons low-sodium grainy mustard

2 teaspoons olive oil

¼ teaspoon dry mustard powder

1 (1-pound) pork tenderloin

2 slices low-sodium whole-wheat bread, crumbled

¼ cup ground walnuts

2 tablespoons cornstarch

**Directions:**

In a small bowl, stir the mustard, olive oil, and mustard powder. Spread this mixture over the pork.

On a plate, mix the bread crumbs, walnuts, and cornstarch. Dip the mustard-coated pork into the crumb -mixture to coat.

Air-fry the pork for 12 to 16 minutes, or until it registers at least 145°F on a meat thermometer. Slice to serve.

**Nutrition:**

Calories: 239

Fat: 9g

Protein: 26g

Carbohydrates: 15g

Sodium: 118mg

Fiber: 2g

Sugar: 3g

# Espresso-Grilled Pork Tenderloin

Preparation time: 15 minutes

Cooking time: 11 minutes

Servings: 4

**Ingredients:**

1 tablespoon packed brown sugar

2 teaspoons espresso powder

1 teaspoon ground paprika

½ teaspoon dried marjoram

1 tablespoon honey

1 tablespoon freshly squeezed lemon juice

2 teaspoons olive oil

1 (1-pound) pork tenderloin

**Directions:**

Mix the brown sugar, espresso powder, paprika, and marjoram in a small bowl.

Stir in the honey, lemon juice, and olive oil until well mixed.

Spread the honey mixture over the pork and let stand for 10 minutes at room temperature.

Roast the tenderloin in the air fryer basket for 9 to 11 minutes, or until the pork registers at least 145°F on a meat thermometer. Slice the meat to serve.

**Nutrition:**

Calories: 177

Fat: 5g

Protein: 23g

Carbohydrates: 10g

Sodium: 61mg

Fiber: 1g

Sugar: 8g

# Pork and Potatoes

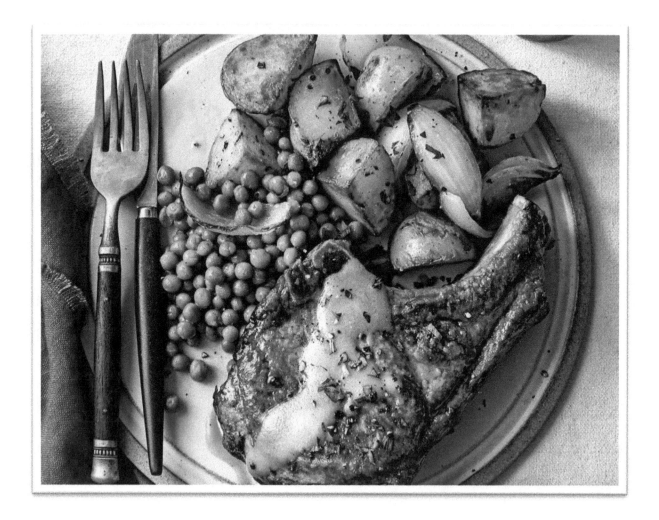

Preparation time: 15 minutes

Cooking time: 25 minutes

Servings: 4

**Ingredients:**

2 cups creamer potatoes, rinsed and dried

2 teaspoons olive oil

1-pound pork tenderloin,1-inch cubes

1 onion, chopped

1 red bell pepper, chopped

2 garlic cloves, minced

½ teaspoon dried oregano

2 tablespoons low-sodium chicken broth

**Directions:**

Toss the potatoes and olive oil to coat in a medium bowl.

Put the potatoes in the air fryer basket—roast for 15 minutes.

In a medium metal bowl, mix the potatoes, pork, onion, red bell pepper, garlic, and oregano.

Drizzle with the chicken broth. Put the bowl in the air fryer basket.

Roast for about 10 minutes more, shaking the basket once during cooking, until the pork reaches at least 145°F on a meat thermometer and the potatoes are tender. Serve immediately.

**Nutrition:**

Calories: 235

Fat: 5g

Protein: 26g

Carbohydrates: 22g

Sodium: 66mg

Fiber: 3g

Sugar: 4g

# Light Herbed Meatballs

Preparation time: 15 minutes

Cooking time: 17 minutes

Servings: 24

**Ingredients:**

1 medium onion, minced

2 garlic cloves, minced

1 teaspoon olive oil

1 slice low-sodium whole-wheat bread, crumbled

3 tablespoons 1 percent milk

1 teaspoon dried marjoram

1 teaspoon dried basil

1-pound 96 percent lean ground beef

**Directions:**

In a 6-by-2-inch pan, combine the onion, garlic, and olive oil. Air-fry for 2 to 4 minutes, or until the vegetables are crisp-tender.

Transfer the vegetables to a medium bowl, and add the bread crumbs, milk, marjoram, and basil. Mix well.

Add the ground beef. With your hands, work the mixture gently but thoroughly until combined. Form the meat mixture into about 24 (1-inch) meatballs.

Bake the meatballs, in batches, in the air fryer basket for 12 to 17 minutes, or until they reach 160°F on a meat thermometer. Serve immediately.

**Nutrition:**

Calories: 190

Fat: 6g

Protein: 25g

Carbohydrates: 8g

Sodium: 120mg

Fiber: 1g

Sugar: 2g

# Brown Rice and Beef-Stuffed Bell Peppers

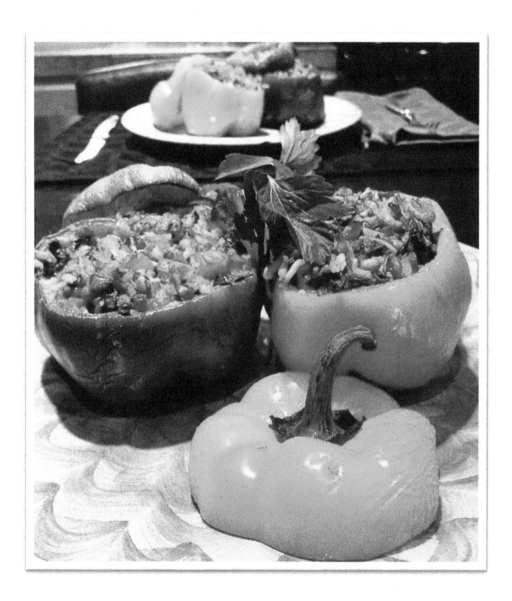

Preparation time: 15 minutes

Cooking time: 16 minutes

Servings: 4

**Ingredients:**

4 medium bell peppers, any colors, rinsed, tops removed

1 medium onion, chopped

½ cup grated carrot

2 teaspoons olive oil

2 medium beefsteak tomatoes, chopped

1 cup cooked brown rice

1 cup chopped cooked low-sodium roast beef (see Tip)

1 teaspoon dried marjoram

**Directions:**

Remove the stems from the bell pepper tops and chop the tops.

In a 6-by-2-inch pan, combine the chopped bell pepper tops, onion, carrot, and olive oil — Cook for 2 to 4 minutes, or until the vegetables are crisp-tender.

Transfer the vegetables to a medium bowl. Add the -tomatoes, brown rice, roast beef, and marjoram. Stir to mix.

Stuff the vegetable mixture into the bell peppers. Place the bell peppers in the air fryer basket.

Bake for 11 to 16 minutes, or until the peppers are tender and the filling is hot. Serve immediately.

**Nutrition:**

Calories: 206

Fat: 6g

Protein: 18g

Carbohydrates: 20g

Sodium: 105mg

Fiber: 3g

Sugar: 5g

# Beef and Broccoli

Preparation time: 15 minutes

Cooking time: 18 minutes

Servings: 4

**Ingredients:**

2 tablespoons cornstarch

½ cup low-sodium beef broth

1 teaspoon low-sodium soy sauce

12 ounces sirloin strip steak, cut into 1-inch cubes

2½ cups broccoli florets

1 onion, chopped

1 cup sliced cremini mushrooms

1 tablespoon grated fresh ginger

Brown rice, cooked (optional)

**Directions:**

In a medium bowl, stir the cornstarch, beef broth, and soy sauce.

Add the beef and toss to coat. Let stand for 5 minutes at room temperature.

With a slotted spoon, transfer the beef from the broth mixture into a medium metal bowl. Reserve the broth.

Add the broccoli, onion, mushrooms, and ginger to the beef. Place the bowl into the air fryer and cook for 12 to 15 minutes or until the beef reaches at least 145°F on a meat thermometer, and the vegetables are tender.

Add the reserved broth and cook for 2 to 3 minutes more, or until the sauce boils.

Serve over hot cooked brown rice.

**Nutrition:**

Calories: 240

Fat: 6g

Protein: 19g

Carbohydrates: 11g

Sodium: 107mg

Fiber: 2g

Sugar: 3g

# Beef and Fruit Stir-Fry

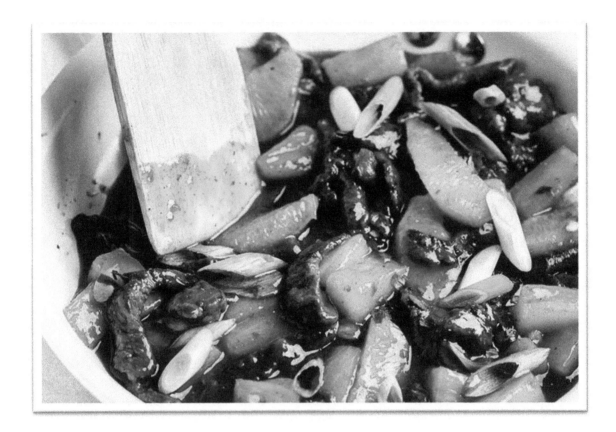

Preparation time: 15 minutes

Cooking time: 11 minutes

Servings: 4

**Ingredients:**

12 ounces sirloin tip steak, thinly sliced

1 tablespoon freshly squeezed lime juice

1 cup canned mandarin orange segments, drained, liquid reserved

1 cup canned pineapple chunks, drained, liquid reserved

1 teaspoon low-sodium soy sauce

1 tablespoon cornstarch

1 teaspoon olive oil

2 scallions, white and green parts, sliced

Brown rice, cooked (optional)

**Directions:**

In a medium bowl, mix the steak with the lime juice. Set aside.

In a small bowl, thoroughly mix 3 tablespoons of reserved mandarin orange juice, 3 tablespoons of reserved pineapple juice, the soy sauce, and cornstarch.

Drain the beef and transfer it to a medium metal bowl, reserving the juice. Stir the reserved liquid into the mandarin-pineapple juice mixture. Set aside.

Add the olive oil and scallions to the steak. Place the metal bowl in the air fryer, cook for 3 to 4 minutes, and shake the basket once cooking.

Stir in the mandarin oranges, pineapple, and juice -mixture. Cook for 3 to 7 minutes more, or until the sauce is bubbling and the beef is tender and reaches at least 145°F on a meat thermometer.

Stir and serve over hot cooked brown rice, if desired.

**Nutrition:**

Calories: 212

Fat: 4g

Protein: 19g

Carbohydrates: 28g

Sodium: 105mg

Fiber: 2g

Sugar: 22g

# Beef Risotto

Preparation time: 15 minutes

Cooking time: 24 minutes

Servings: 4

**Ingredients:**

2 teaspoons olive oil

1 onion, finely chopped

3 garlic cloves, minced

½ cup chopped red bell pepper

¾ cup short-grain rice

1¼ cups low-sodium beef broth

½ cup (about 3 ounces) chopped cooked roast beef (see Tip)

3 tablespoons grated Parmesan cheese

**Directions:**

In a 6-by-2-inch pan, combine the olive oil, onion, garlic, and red bell pepper. Place the pan in the air fryer for 2 -minutes, or until the vegetables are crisp-tender. Remove from the air fryer.

Add the rice, beef broth, and roast beef. Return the pan to the air fryer and bake for 18 to 22 minutes, stirring once during cooking, until the rice is tender and the beef reaches at least 145°F on a meat thermometer.

Remove the pan from the air fryer. Stir in the Parmesan cheese, then serve.

**Nutrition:**

Calories: 227

Fat: 5g

Protein: 10g

Carbohydrates: 33g

Sodium: 88mg

Fiber: 2g

CPSIA information can be obtained
at www.ICGtesting.com
Printed in the USA
BVHW060843180321
602885BV00011B/1121

9 781801 445276